Tendonitis and the different types of tendonitis explained.

Tendonitis Symptoms, Diagnosis, Treatment Options, Stretches and Exercises all included.

by

Rowan Beetson

Published by IMB Publishing 2013

Table Of Contents

Table of Contents

Table of Contents

Table of Contents

Table of Contents

Foreword

This book pledges to excite readers, as well as to be an assemblage of knowledge accessible to any individual who is aiming at understanding tendonitis as a condition, its epidemiology, pathophysiology, progression course, existing kinds and their managements.
Rowan has exceptionally excelled at addressing the most commonly asked questions on tendonitis, thus catering to the needs of the reader, which is the intention of any book.

This book offers readers eye-opening views, tips and exercise techniques aimed at an optimal well-being of mental and physical states for a healthy lifestyle.

Acknowledgements

For their contributions to this book, this token of appreciation goes to:
Jacob S. Smith
Ronald Cunty
Donovan Slovak
Carla Brown
Celestine Schuss
Bianca Murphy

And

My family.

Introduction

Tendonitis is a common enfeebling condition, which is estimated to be affecting tens of thousands of workers by the Bureau of Labor Statistics, and is also a common reason for doctor's visits. It results in a significant deficit in activity and in long-term loss of productivity if not treated early and adequately.

The term tendonitis is used interchangeably with tendinitis. It is derived from two words: *tendon* - a fibrous band which connects a muscle to a bone, allowing the pulling force of muscle contraction to be transferred to a bone, bringing about locomotion - and *–itis* - a Latin suffix meaning inflammation. Research for decades goes against the notion that inflammation of a tendon is the primary culprit cause of tendonitis, but rather of *tendinosis*. The use of these terms can be confusing, though altogether different. Tendinosis, derived from *tendon* and *-osis,* the latter implying a change within an organ, associated with degeneration without inflammation. Tendinosis is thus a cellular derangement of makeup components of the tendon, in particular collagen - a type of protein that gives tendons their structure of multiple thick fibers intertwined together. Losing elasticity and strength renders them vulnerable to *Repeated Stress Injuries (RSIs)* with partial or total rupture in severe cases. This is actually the reason why corticosteroid injections give temporary relief on tendonitis, as it is not merely inflammation. The *American Medical Association - ICD-9* code, though to be replaced by the *ICD-10* code, presents this debilitating condition as tendinosis interchangeably with tendinopathy.

The *American Association for Orthopaedic Surgeons* (AAOS) classifies tendinopathies by how they are viewed under the microscope, which facilitates a logical approach to treatment as it depicts the underlying etiology. Etiology being listed as multi-factorial, including biochemical changes resulting from intrinsic tendon protein degeneration (hypocellular, vascular and nervous ingrowths, necrosis and calcification) to atrophic degeneration (ageing, microtrauma, and vascular compromise).

This book is thus a revelation of an inside story of tendonitis, with tendinosis lurking in the background, in understandable terms outlining insightful knowledge, to educate the reader.

The author is a retired sports medicine professor, who has experience with tendonitis in all of its forms - rotator cuff, Achilles tendonitis, golfer's elbow, tennis elbow, jumper's knee amongst others. He has placed some efforts on elaborating tendinosis as a stressing medical condition, evidenced by the impact it has on the general public; given the growing prevalence of tendonitis because of sporting activity extension in older age groups. Updates and re-evaluation of diagnosis, pathophysiology, etiology and treatment plans of tendonitis have long been overdue. Unveil tendonitis in this exceptional educative guide.

Common abbreviations used in text

ABI	Autologous blood injection
ACL	Anterior cruciate ligament
ART	Active release technique
CRP	C-reactive protein
CT-scan	Computer tomography
DJD	Degenerative joint disease
ECM	Extracellular matrix
ESR	Erythrocyte sedimentation rate
FBC	Full blood count
FBP	Full blood picture
FROM	Full range of motion
ICD	International classification of diseases
LCL	Lateral collateral ligament
MCL	Medial collateral ligament
MRI	Magnetic resonance imaging
NSAIDs	Non-steroidal anti-inflammatory drugs
PCL	Posterior cruciate ligament
PRP	Protein-rich plasma
RICE	Rest, ice, compression, and elevation
RSIs	Repeated stress injuries
3D	Three-dimensional

Chapter 1) Tendon

1) What is a tendon?

A *tendon* (or *sinew*) is a tough, yet flexible, band of fibrous connective tissue that connects muscle to bone and is capable of withstanding tension. Think of it as an intermediary between muscles and bones. The Achilles tendon, one that you've most probably heard of, was named after a Greek demigod hero who suffered the tendon's fatal weakness. Similar to tendons are *ligaments* and *fasciae*, as they are all connective tissues made from collagen protein - although ligaments connect bone to bone while fasciae muscle to muscle. All of these connective tissue types, including bone, nerves, and blood vessels, are part of the musculoskeletal system.

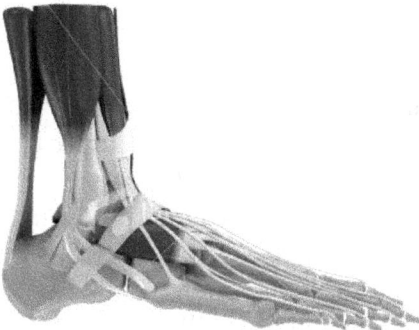

Tendons are pure white in color with a fibrous, yet elastic, texture. Their shapes and sizes differ by location within the human body, having rounded cords, at times are flat ribbon–like, and/or appear striped. The great tensile strength of tendons, which is necessary to resist stress generated by muscle activity, is made possible by the large quantity of collagen fibers intertwined together to form remarkably thick, tough and strong ropes. People usually only mention collagen as a component of tendons because it occupies a high percentage of the dry mass of normal tendons at 86% and is considered to be the standard unit of a tendon. Besides collagen, a tendon consists of 70% water and other constituents located within the space around collagen fibers- the so-called *extracellular matrix* (ECM), which includes cells (*tenocytes, tenoblasts, chondrocytes)*, a stretchable protein called *elastin*, elements such as copper, manganese, and calcium, also *proteoglycans*, which are organic substances, and *glycoproteins*. Proteoglycans are hydrophilic molecules that enable water-soluble substances to dissolve fast in the tendon and aid the transport of cells. Glycoproteins are structural pillars that act as adhesives, which participate in tendon repair and regeneration. Some other important proteins, like *teniscin-C,* should be mentioned because of their role at the muscle-tendon junction and the bone-tendon junction. Besides, they also play a role as an elastic component and aid to align and orient collagen fibers. Tenoblasts found in the ECM are immature tenocytes, which bear a spindle shape with vast cytoplasmic organelles showing their high metabolic activity. Tenocytes, however, have a low number of cytoplasmic organelles portraying a reduced metabolic process and are responsible for the production of collagen. Tenocyte energy generation, like many other body cells, is driven by oxygen in the *Krebs cycle*, but they have an added advantage of being capable to produce energy in the absence of oxygen (*anaerobically*) and by yet another alternative energy-producing process known as *the pentose phosphate pathway*. It is by this that tendons can withstand high tension for long periods of time without suffering ischemia or necrosis. In total, all of these components just prove how tendons are simple, yet complex.

2) What exactly is collagen?

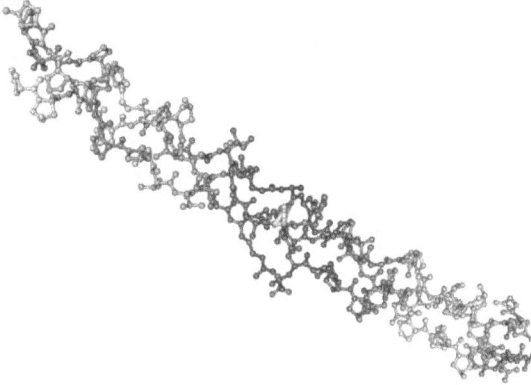

Collagen is the most abundant protein in mammals, including humans, accounting for approximately 30% of the total protein content of the human body. It is usually termed *"body glue."* It is the glue that holds body tissues together and is found in fibrous tissues such as skin, tendons, ligaments, fasciae, bones, blood vessels, and even intestines. Collagen is vital for strength, shape and elasticity of tissues like tendons without which movement is not possible.

The building blocks of collagen are amino acids, since it is a protein and therefore its main elements are hydrogen, oxygen, nitrogen and carbon. This structure makes collagen vulnerable to weak acids or alkalis and heat, which is why boiling meat makes it soft enough for digestion. The arrangement of amino acids in collagen and connections between them may differ, forming the different kinds of collagen. 29 distinct collagens are present in animal tissue, with genetic selection responsible for their distribution in tissues from species to species. In the human body, type I collagen is the most abundant, covering over 90% of all the collagen in the body. It is found in tendons, bones, skin and ligaments. Other types of collagen may still be present in these tissues but in small quantities. For instance, besides abundant type

I collagen in tendons, types II, III, V, X also are present in meager quantities.

Tenocytes produce collagen molecules, which aggregate end-to-end and side-to-side to form collagen fibrils. These fibrils are similar in structure and conglomerate in threes to form a triple helical 3D structure of collagen, *tropocollagen*. The triple helical fibers are covered by a protective sheath of a reticular connective tissue network known as *endotenon*, forming even larger bundles of collagen called *fascicles*. A great number of these fascicles are covered by yet another sheath, the *epitenon*, to form the tendon. Blood and lymphatic vessels, together with nerves, enter and leave the tendon via the *paratenon* sustaining its viability. Some tendons, especially those found in areas of increased mechanical stress, e.g. fingers, are covered by an outer *synovial sheath*, which has a *synovial membrane* that produces *synovial fluid*. Synovial fluid is a lubricant- like oil is to a bicycle chain, allowing smooth and friction-free tendon mobility.

With age the production of collagen begins to slow down and tissues begin to lose their strength and structure, as such skin becomes fragile, less elastic, and wrinkles set in, joints lose their flexibility, hair its color, tendons degenerate, become weak and susceptible to RSIs- causing tendonitis. It is by this that collagen as a substance is used in cosmetic treatment for wrinkles, wound care managements and burn surgery.

3) Tendon physiology

Tendons, while generally known as structures which transmit muscle contraction to bones, are categorized into 2 main types: positional tendons, such as hand tendons, which are stiff, serving a positional maintenance purpose; and the other type, weight-bearing tendons, which are more elastic and flexible, where the Achilles tendon is an example. As a larger portion of the general population takes part in physical and recreational activities, annually the frequency of tendon injuries is on the increase as well as health care costs and patient morbidity.

Tendon physiology aims to understand how its components interact and work together at a molecular and functional basis giving the whole integrated behavior of a tendon. We understand that all living tissues have a nervous supply, blood vessels, mechanisms by which to function and a repair strategy in case of injury. Tendons are no exception.

a) Blood supply

Tendon blood supply consists of 3 main sources, the largest being extrinsic blood vessels travelling in the paratenon. The other 2 sources are intrinsic blood vessels from the muscles and bones. The ratios of blood being supplied by the intrinsic source to that from the extrinsic vary from tendon to tendon.

The tendon is a fibrous band, which connects muscle to bone. As it is an intermediate, this requires it to be connected to either component. At the *myotendinous junction* vascular branches from the muscle continue between the collagen fascicles of the tendon. However, these vessels cover approximately a third of the tendon from the junction. At the insertion point of a tendon to bone, the *osteotendinous junction,* periosteal blood vessels spill over to supply part of the tendon, though this supply is limited. Bones are covered by a thick fibrous connective tissue called the *periosteum*, blood vessels from which spillover occurs to supply the tendon. This arrangement of blood supply to the tendon leaves the tendon centre regions with minimal blood supply, the so-called *watershed zone.* Therefore, the watershed zone of a tendon is part of the tendon that has the weakest blood supply. Also, zones of maximum torsion, friction or compression have a compromised vascular supply. These hypovascular zones are of importance because they are the most prone to injury.

At the osteotendinous junction the tendon attaches to bone at a 90-degree angle in four layers. The tendon collagen fibers, as they appear in the tendon, then become fibro-cartilaginous in texture as they transition to bone. *Sharpey's fibers* originate in the bone and end in the periosteum. These make sure that when the tendon enters the bone it is imbedded rather than ingrown into the bone tissues and is continuous with it.

For tendons that are encircled by a synovial sheath, blood vessels through the *vincula* reach the inside of the synovial sheath where they form a vascular network known as a *plexus* that supplies the superficial part of the tendon. In the absence of a synovial sheath the paratenon covers that job. Also, synovial fluid acts as a source of nutrients as they diffuse from within this fluid into the tendon.

b) Innervation

Tendon innervation originates from the musculo-tendinous junction, where myelinated nerve fibers cross to enter the endotenous sheath. In the paratenon, nerves form a plexus whose branches penetrate to the epitenon. Encapsulated myelinated nerve fiber groups called *Golgi tendon organs* are localized more at the muscle insertion site and function to detect tendon tension levels, the so-called *mechanoreceptors*. In a tendon, both sympathetic and parasympathetic nerve supplies exist. Unmyelinated nerve endings, *nociceptors*, give sensory signals to pain, temperature and proprioception. All these nerves are more at the tendon surface and consist of afferents only.

c) Biomechanics

Tendon strength is related to its thickness and collagen fiber quantity such that an area of 1 square centimeter is capable of withstanding tensional stress from a 500-1000 kg weight. Tendons transmit forces from muscle to bone and absorb external forces to limit muscle damage. They exhibit such high levels of mechanical strength, elasticity and excellent flexibility adequate to perform their role. They display *stress relaxation* and *creep*. What does that mean? The mechanical behaviors of tendons depend on the quantity of collagen fibers, their fiber types and interfiber bonds. At rest, collagen fibrils are crimped, that is they are loose and coiled. As they begin to be stretched by a force, the initial strain of which is up to 2% represents flattening of the crimp pattern to a non-weaved position of collagen fibers and fibrils. This initial step is called the *toe phase* and if presented on a graph will be the *toe region*. This initial straightening of tendon collagen fibers has been proven to be the result of molecular elongation. As more tension is exerted on the tendon, it deforms in a linear fashion due to tropocollagen structures sliding over each other to become parallel. At this stage, unlike molecular elongation in the initial stage, gaps between tendon molecules increase, thus stretching and tightening collagen fibers further. If the strain is <4% where tendons can withstand the tensional force, it returns to its original length behaving as a rubber band substance. When strain exceeds 4%, microscopic damage appears, which can accumulate if the process is repeated over and over, resulting in an ultimate tendon injury after a longtime use. This is how tendonitis develops. At strains of 8-10%, macroscopic tendon failure occurs, which results from triple helical structure slippage and breaking. A partial or total tendon rupture results at this point. The fibers at the ruptured ends recoil into a tangled knot.

4) Tendon function

Tendons are tough, fibrous cords of connective tissue that connect skeletal muscles to bones. Basically, without them you couldn't move. Tendons enable free and flexible movement of the body. Running, dancing, swimming and driving are made possible by tendons, not only tendons though, but the complete musculoskeletal system, without which tendons could not function alone. A longer tendon, especially the heel, gives an advantage to the runner and is decided upon by genetics. A tendon can be compared to an elastic band where upon stretching it lengthens and when released recoils back to its original state. As for a tendon, when a muscle contracts, it pulls the tendon with it, thus stretching the tendon, which when it recoils transmits the muscle force to the bone and therefore actively facilitates movement.

One misconception is that the only function of tendons is to connect muscles to bones. This is an understatement because tendons have a high elastic capacity; such that they are flexible and can store and release energy. Also, tendons are an added benefit to muscles. How? The force that a muscle can generate is dependent upon its length. Stretching a tendon also lengthens the muscle, thus increasing the total muscle length and the force that it can generate.

5) Tendinopathies

Tendons are a fundamental component of the contractile unit. Most tendon injuries occur near joints since these areas are the sites of repetitive motion resulting in overuse over a long period of time. Tendon injuries may appear to have occurred suddenly, but that is rarely the case. Often, many tendon micro-tears occur which accumulate over time until the final tendon snap. Achilles tendon, rotator cuff, and tennis or golfer's elbow are among the commonest tendon injuries.

Recent studies have shown that overused tendon pathologies are devoid of inflammatory cells and instead have a disintegrating collagen matrix that is known as tendinosis. *Tendinosis* is therefore the primary culprit to overused tendon injuries. Tendinosis refers to tiny micro-tears around and inside a tendon resulting from overuse of already degenerating tendon components resulting in a less potent structure that is vulnerable to repetitive stress injuries. The term *tendinopathy* is used by medical professionals to mean tendon injuries whether they result from inflammation, degeneration and/or repeated use.

Tenosynovitis is another chronic overused tendon injury, which is irritation and inflammation between a tendon and its synovial sheath. Note that this condition only occurs in tendons that are covered by a synovial sheath such as the long head of the biceps tendon. The sheath is supposed to reduce friction between the tendon and the area that it overlies- where sliding often occurs. Chronic repetitive overloading results in adhesions forming between the tendon and its sheath, subsequently initiating an inflammatory process. The symptoms of tenosynovitis and tendinosis are similar though a distinction can be made between the two. One has to understand whether a tendon has a synovial sheath or not - if it doesn't, then tendinosis is the most probable cause.

Avulsion tendon injuries are acute, occurring with a one-time excessive tension strain onto a tendon, resulting in its attachment to bone being torn off. Tendon avulsion injuries often occur in regions where tendons attach to a relatively small site in relation to the muscle bulk, such as the hamstring muscle attachment.

Calcific tendonitis should be mentioned since it is a relatively common tendinopathy. Calcific tendonitis is a condition that causes the development of calcium deposits in a tendon, which are usually small (about 1-2 centimeter sizes). This occurs more in diabetic patients, but can occur in anyone, often above 40 years of age. The reason as to why tendons calcify is not clear, but it is thought that delayed healing contributes. Normally when a tendon heals, fibroblasts produce collagen. A cell swap occurs for *osteoblasts*, bone-producing cells resulting in growth of bone (calcium) in the tendon. The course of calcific tendonitis is unpredictable, resolving spontaneously without surgery. Three phases of calcific tendonitis are known: the pre-calcific, calcific and post-calcific phases. At the pre-calcific phase, no signs appear, but the cellular changes are occurring in the background. The calcific phase is marked by calcium excretion from cells, forming calcium deposits. These deposits appear white like chalk. All of these processes are pain-free. A resting period follows where no further calcium deposits appear. Pain is experienced when these calcium deposits begin to be reabsorbed, appearing like toothpaste in color and consistency. The post-calcific phase denotes disappearance of any calcium deposits from the tendon, thus appearing normal.

Tears may occur in tendons. If they occur in ligaments, they are called *sprains*, and if in muscles they are called *strains*. *Tendon tears* can be graded, mild or 1st degree, moderate to severe or 2nd degree, and 3rd degree being a complete rupture. Tendon tears disrupt muscle function and they lose the ability to transmit muscle contraction forces to bone, and therefore the bone is not moved as required. The *extensor mechanism* of the leg as an example, the thigh muscle (quadriceps) is attached to the kneecap by the quadriceps tendon and to the shin bone by the patella tendon. If at any point on these tendons there is a complete break, the extension function will seize and a patient will not be able to extend the leg at the knee.

Tendon injuries often occur in people who play particular sports such as baseball, football, gymnastics, volleyball, running and tennis, but jobs which require one to be having a repetitive motion of some sort like typing, overhead stretching, and carrying heavy loads can also result in tendon injuries. Sporting activities that require a sudden start e.g. jumps or sprints might cause an injury upon takeoff - the abrupt tension strain may be too much for the tendon to handle, resulting in it giving way.

Dr Nirschl is one of the founding members of the United States Tennis Association Sports Science Committee. It is of importance to mention that Dr. Nirschl is known worldwide for his extensive research on tendon injuries. He proposed four stages of tendinopathy. These stages are the ones often used by specialists as tendon injury grading to assist in treatment plan choice.

Stage 0: The tendon is healthy with no signs of inflammation. Histological examination reveals collagen fibers and fibrils to be well organized and no blood cells exist within the tendon. The tendon is firm, non-tender with a normal temperature.

Stage 1: Acute tendonitis - the tendon degeneration is symptomatic with pain, swelling, tenderness, warmth and reduced function. Histological examination reveals micro-tears with inflammatory cells and collagen fiber configurations are distorted.

Stage 2: Chronic tendonitis - even more pronounced tendon degeneration and vascular compromise. Histology shows more micro-tears, more inflammatory cells and collagen fiber disorientation. A sufferer does not use the limb due to chronic pain, which is accompanied by severe tenderness.

Stage 3: Tendinosis - intra-tendon degeneration occurs due to repetitive stress injuries, cellular and tissue aging, together with hypovascularity. Histology reveals hypercellularity, regional necrosis and collagen disorganization. Tendon is palpable and large with swelling of tissues and the tendon sheath may also be swollen with or without pain.

Stage 4: Rupture - tendon fails to withstand tensional forces, collagen fibers are totally disrupted and broken. The muscle is weak and painful. A patient is unable to use the affected limb.

a) Symptoms

Tendinopathies have symptoms that are almost always the same, regardless of the tendon in question. Pain along the site of the tendon location is the main complaint of patients e.g. for Achilles tendon the pain is along the back of the foot- especially upon stretching by tiptoes. In tendinosis the pain is mild to moderate though may worsen suddenly, causing so-called flare-ups. A flare-up is a sudden increase in intensity of pain on an already symptomatic tendon. This does not mean that the condition has worsened or the tendon has ruptured, it is just a concentrated form of the already existing pathology due maybe to a long repetitive activity prior to its occurrence, such as a long drive. Tenderness, swelling, redness, stiffness, a popping sound and temporary reflex non-use of a muscle, what is known as *pseudo-paralysis*, are other symptoms which are presented by patients with tendinopathies, not necessarily that all have to be present at once.

b) Diagnosis

Diagnosis of tendon injuries should be done by a physician and/or a specialist like an orthopaedic specialist or sports medicine specialist. Physical examination is always required to rule out any other *differential diagnosis* conditions. Differential diagnosis is of great importance and ranges from a wide spectrum of candidate diseases. It could be that bones, ligaments, bursae, muscles, joints and neurovascular structures of a particular region in close proximity to the tendon are injured instead. Differential diagnosis will rule out any immediate medical emergencies that may require early medical intervention, such as decompressing a septic joint. Other investigations can be ordered by a physician that may consist of laboratory *blood works* and/or imaging. Blood work is a term used to mean any medical blood test performed to check for any component of blood. In tendon injuries the most commonly tested are *full blood picture* (FBP), *C-reactive protein* (CRP), and *erythrocyte sedimentation rate* (ESR). Full blood picture at times is called full blood count (FBC), and measures the cellular components of blood which are pointers to certain ongoing processes in the body - for instance, an increase in white blood cells may mean an infection. An ESR test is done to check the time in which a drop of blood reaches the bottom of a water-filled test tube. In inflammation, blood cells are coated by inflammatory substances, thus making them heavy and fast to reach the bottom. This too is a differential disease clue generator and/or supporter. C-reactive protein is considered to be the primary protein produced by the liver as a response to inflammation and/or an infection. The higher the CRP, the greater the probability that some inflammatory process is going on somewhere in the body. All these blood works are used for differential diagnosis.

Imaging such as X-rays, ultrasound, MRI and CT-scan can be performed. X-rays, being cheap and readily available in many medical centers, are the frequent imaging done for differential diagnosis. Pathologies in bones are visualized, and also if a tendon has some calcifications they too can be seen. Ultrasound is important to differentiate conditions such as fluid accumulation in a joint or muscle forming cysts and/or abscesses, but in tendon injuries can be confirmatory as they can show tendon tears. Their limitation in use is on obese patients whose tissues are too deep for the ultrasound resolution power. Magnetic resonance imaging (MRI) is a specialized expensive medical test that uses a large magnetic field to generate images on a screen or display. MRI has a higher resolution capacity so that even the smallest of the micro-tendon tears can be visualized, including pathologies in blood supply such as infracts. This makes it the imaging test of choice for most, if not all, tendinopathies. Computer

Tomographies, CT-scans, are not as effective on soft tissues as MRI is, but are excellent for bone pathologies where even the slightest change in blood supply can be captured.

c) Treatment options

As painful as they may be, good news is that mild to moderate tendon injuries can heal on their own, third-degree injuries however require surgery. Tendon healing is a very slow process owing to their low metabolic rate and poor blood supply of the regions often injured, though the healing process can be somewhat sped up by self-intervening and/or medical/physiotherapy as a means of tendon injury rehabilitation. Other treatment plans include:

a) The *RICE method*; it is commonly used and many people use it without even knowing its name. The RICE method is important and easy to follow and a patient or sufferer can initiate it by themselves at home. RICE stands for rest, ice, compression and elevation. Rest the affected area e.g. in Achilles tendonitis, avoid putting weight on the leg of the affected side. One might even need crutches or in rotator cuff tendinosis carrying heavy things and letting the shoulder free should be avoided. A splint, brace and/or sling should be used as a temporary immobilizer. Ice has been shown to reduce inflammation by cooling off the affected area since the inflammatory process results in local heat emission. However, ice should never be placed in direct contact with the skin because it can cause a thermal burn. Cover the ice with a towel or cloth before placing it in contact with skin and/or use a bag of frozen vegetables. Swelling is one of the symptoms in tendon injuries; it further compromises blood supply by compressing on small tissue vessels. This increases local tissue ischemia and worsening of the condition. Elevate the limb to enhance gravitational lymphatic fluid and blood drainage from the limb, thus reducing swelling. Prop the arm or leg on a pillow to achieve this. Compression using elastic stockings is encouraged as it prevents swelling and at the same time acts as a prophylactic measure to deep vein thrombosis especially in patients with vascular occlusive diseases and systemic ones such as diabetes mellitus.

b) Painkillers are essential to stop the excruciating tendon pain. Rarely are narcotic analgesics used such as morphine. *Non-steroidal anti-inflammatory drugs* (*NSAIDs*) are the main stay for this purpose. They are effective and tolerated by most patients. NSAIDs such as naproxen, ibuprofen, Advil and Motril are available as over-the-counter medications. These drugs do have side effects such as nausea, peptic ulcer disease and increased risk of bleeding. They should be used as short courses occasionally and not long-term unless your physician says otherwise. Prolonged use heightens the probability of adverse effect development. It is still important to get a prescription from your doctor to get the correct best drug choice on the market at the correct doses. Some individuals have allergies to these medications, which should be discovered by your physician when discussing your history and hence a substitute drug for pain relief can be given.

c) Corticosteroid injections, such as cortisone, can be injected at the tendon attachment site. The catch is that the shot has to be in exactly the right spot. Corticosteroids relieve inflammation and thus pain. However, their use is controversial as some specialists argue that pain is a physiological response to injury. If pain is eliminated, the body is kind of tricked to believe that all is well when there is actually an ongoing process. This will lead to worsening of the injury as the body will not respond as it normally should in such situations - for instance, reflex non-use (pseudo paralysis). One will continue using the pain-free limb, further damaging the tendon. Corticosteroid injection side effects include loss of skin pigmentation at the site of injection, tendon atrophy and tendon rupture. Some myths associated with cortisone injections are that the shot is very painful. This is not true, but to some extent there ought to be some pain. Injections will give a prickly pain and since cortisone is not injected alone, it is given together with an anaesthetic medication like Novocain. It is this Novocain which stings and is even more painful than the steroid itself. Another myth is that these injections will lead to muscle bulk development. This is also not true, since the steroids that athletes sometimes use are of a different group - the anabolic steroids are the ones to cause this effect. Cortisone injections are also thought to weaken the bone and tendons. The dose of steroid in this injection is too minimal to elicit such bone changes, but might in tendons because there are local injections at high doses and/or consecutive steroid injections over a short period of time. This is why 3 corticosteroid injections are only allowed to be given in one particular area over 3-4 weeks.

d) Corticosteroid injections are not the only medications used in such a way. Botulism toxin, what is known as Botox, can also be used and/or *autologous blood injection (ABI)* and *platelet-rich plasma injections (PRP)*. Botox is a toxin that when injected at the tendon insertion site causes temporary paralysis of the muscle at the junction. This effect is thought to be useful in resting the tendon to allow for healing. ABI use is based on the theory that blood as a living tissue consists of cells, hormones, nutrients, electrolytes and elements that are essential for metabolism and growth. If injected into an injured tendon, these growth factors boost the healing process. In PRP only the liquid component of blood is used. This liquid component, called *plasma,* constitutes all the growth substances except cells. It acts in the same way as the ABI. ABI and PRP are given once or twice, though if ineffective are rarely given thrice; a substitute treatment plan is initiated.

e) *Prolotherapy* is yet another injectable type of tendon treatment, where an irritant such as glucose is injected into the tendon. This causes a local tendon reaction associated with production of more fibrous substances and tendon thickening. This increases healing and together with physiotherapy has been shown to be an effective treatment modality.

f) Ultrasound and *shockwaves* may be used as pain relief treatment therapies. High-energy shockwaves are passed through the skin overlying a tendon, and ultrasound emits non-audible waves that reach the tendon and relieve pain. These two therapies require multiple sessions for their effect to be appreciated e.g. a 10-minute session 5 times a week.

g) *Active release technique* (ART) can be used on joints. It is thought that tendons over time develop adhesions, which restrict movement and cause pain. In ART, under anesthesia a physician breaks these adhesions, acquiring full range of motion (FROM) after which physiotherapy is aggressively implemented to prevent redevelopment of adhesions and to maintain the newly attained FROM.

h) Natural treatment modalities are also used and these include herbal substances such as curcumin and St. John's Wort, salts ferrum phos and Silicea, acupuncture, exercises and homeopathy. Diet can also be used to supplement for nutrients, for instance omega 3 found in fish oils, walnuts, omega-3-enriched dairy products and flax seeds. Omega-3 has for been known for a long time to reduce inflammation and its anti-inflammatory makes it an important food source.

i) When conservative treatment fails, surgery is indicated. Surgery is also indicated to torn tendons. Surgery is specific for the tendon pathology under treatment. For inflammatory processes, debridement is performed, which constitutes removal of the affected part of the tendon. Detaching and reattaching a tendon may also be done e.g. in tennis or golfer's elbow surgery. Other surgical procedures involve creating space for the compressed tendons to be free, an example being acromioplasty in rotator cuff tendonitis. End-to-end suturing can be performed to partially or totally torn tendons. These procedures can be open surgery and/or scopic types where a camera fiber-optic device is used through a small hole to visualize the tendon under repair.

6) Tendon repair

After injury tendons are required to regenerate broken fibers and fibrils and to restore the sliding mechanisms over its surroundings, especially tendons that have a synovial sheath.

Initial tendon repair consists of scar tissue formation to provide tendon continuity. However, this scar produces adhesions of the tendon to the surrounding tissues. This prevents normal tendon function. Although rest is necessary for an injured tendon to heal, mobility is of utmost importance to prevent adhesion formation and to increase strength of the tendon. Like bone, a tendon's strength lies in the load in which it carries. This is true even in healing. For a tendon to achieve adequate power it has to be loaded by exercise, though gradual weight increase is recommended since an abrupt overload will further damage a healing tendon.

Tendon healing is composed of two mechanisms. The intrinsic healing mechanism consists of cells migrating from the paratenon to the injured site, whereas the extrinsic mechanism involves cells migrating from injured vessels outside the tendon to the injured site. The true repair process constitutes of both mechanisms and is dependent on many factors including tendon motion post injury and the severity of the injury. The extrinsic tendon healing is known to be the major contributor to adhesion formation while the intrinsic causes rearrangement of collagen fibers at the remodeling phase. These repair mechanisms occur in phases through three stages of tissue inflammation, cell proliferation and remodeling.

a) Tissue inflammation

Soon after injury, disrupted blood vessels bleed and the physiology makeup of the human body is in such a way that any bleeding activates blood clotting factors to form a clot as a way of stopping bleeding. This formed hematoma in turn activates many substances including pro-inflammatory and vessel-dilating substances. Dilated vessels are hyper–permeable, allowing blood cells, such as red blood cells, white blood cells, and platelets, to migrate towards the injured site, which in the usual state is not possible. These cells begin to produce specific chemicals to attract other cells of their kind, and white cells, especially macrophages, engulf dead tissues and debris. *Fibroblasts* are also recruited from blood and these cells secrete extracellular matrix components. Vessel-enhancing factors are also released and initiate formation of new vascular networks, what is known as *angiogenesis*. The formed matrix establishes continuity of the tendon and provides slight stability at the tendon injury site.

b) Cell proliferation

Proliferation is a continuous process of cellular multiplication. Fibroblasts at this phase rapidly proliferate at the injury site and are responsible for the production of more collagen, proteoglycans and extracellular matrix components. Unlike in a normal tendon where ECM and collagen fibers are orderly arranged, a healing tendon has them randomly placed. Instead of the usual type I collagen fibers, type III are produced. By the end of this proliferation stage the injured tendon site consists of extensive ECM with numerous cells and the wound appears to be plugged by a scar-like tissue.

c) Remodeling

At this stage ECM production decreases and so does the cellular content. Type III collagen fibers are replaced by type I fibers. These are arranged along the tendon axis and increase on mechanical strength of the regenerating tendon. This occurs 6-8 weeks after the initial tendon injury. With later times, the collagen fibers interact to form even stronger bonds in an attempt to attain what once was the tendon configuration. However, the resulting tendon strength is never as potent as the initial pre-injury strength.

Chapter 2) Tendonitis

1) Definition

In the body, tendons come in different shapes and sizes. They can be as large as the Achilles tendon and/or small like the tendons of the hand. Regardless of their shape, size and location, in a normal individual, tendons glide easily over a surface when pulled by a contracting muscle. In certain scenarios these tendons become inflamed due to many reasons and the contracting muscle pull becomes irritating and painful. When this impairment occurs, it is called *tendonitis*. A literal translation of tendonitis will be inflammation of a tendon.

Tendonitis is a type of tendinopathy that can occur anywhere in the body where tendons connect muscle to bone, but certain types of tendonitis are more frequent than others. In the upper and lower limbs tendonitis is common in comparison to in the torso and the hip. The most common are shoulder, elbow, knee, heel and the base of the thumb. Tendonitis is named by the affected region - for instance, shoulder tendonitis or elbow tendonitis. Layman terms are also used in naming different kinds of tendonitis by the specific group of people who commonly develop their symptoms, e.g. swimmer's shoulder for shoulder tendonitis, tennis elbow for lateral elbow tendonitis, golfer's elbow, jumper's knee, and many more.

2) Epidemiology

Tendonitis is a common debilitating condition that reduces productivity and affects both males and females at a 1:1 ratio. It can affect anyone, but more so adults over 40 years of age. People who do a lot of recreational sporting activities are often affected, especially if their sporting techniques lack biomechanical body position control. This per se does not mean that tendonitis develops due to poor sporting technique as the myth has it, but that poor technique is one of the risk factors to developing tendonitis, which is an overuse injury. People who work in positions that require repetitive motion, like typists, meat cutters, and gardeners, are at risk of developing tendonitis. The elderly are also susceptible because with age our tendons lose elasticity and extracellular matrix components degenerate, making them weak and vulnerable to repetitive stress injuries.

3) Risk factors

Risk factors are things that increase the probability or likelihood of developing a disease or condition. For example, obesity significantly increases the risk of developing hypertension and/or hypertensive heart disease. Thus, obesity is a risk factor for hypertension and heart disease.

Tendonitis also has risk factors that heighten its development; they are divided into intrinsic and extrinsic factors. Intrinsic factors consist of congenital or acquired deformities such as limb length discrepancies, muscular insufficiency, muscle imbalance, and/or body misalignments like in scoliosis. Extrinsic factors include training surfaces, the equipment and footwear used during sport, and training errors such as technique and fatigue. Other factors are as follows:

a) Sex
Males predominate in tendon injuries, Achilles tendon for one at a ratio 7:1 with women. However, more women in recent decades are participating in physical activities as a result of weight loss programs, for example, so their percentage of tendonitis is also on the rise.

b) Age
Tendons degenerate with age; over-40s are susceptible to tendonitis with a peak range between 40-60 years of age. In children, tendons are very strong in comparison to their immature growing skeletons, so that high energy injuries often affect their growth plates, leaving tendons intact. Osgood-Schlatter disease is by far the only common tendon pathology in active children. It consists of tendon pain and irritation on the area just below the

knee, on the front side of the leg where the patella tendon inserts into the shin bone.

c) Sports
Sporting activities that have repetitive motions are included tennis, baseball, swimming, basketball, golf, running, javelin, long or high jump, etc.

d) Specific jobs
Jobs that involve being in awkward positions for a long time, frequent overhead reaching, vibration and repetitive movements are on the forefront. Examples are gardening, shoveling, painting, scrubbing, carpentry and raking.

e) Concomitant diseases, especially metabolic ones, where diabetes mellitus is top listed and collagen production pathologies. Rheumatoid arthritis is another systemic condition that affects tendons frequently.

4) Causes

Tendonitis results from a tendon injury, for example at takeoff during a sprint, but most commonly occurs gradually over time due to micro-trauma, RSIs that accumulate and do not adequately heal. The bad news is that tendonitis occurs in *"watershed zones,"* where oxygen and nutrients are at their minimal distribution, which delays healing. Occasionally there can be an anatomical tendonitis. This kind is common at the shoulder, e.g. where the supraspinatus tendon is impinged, resulting in its irritation and progression to a tendonitis. In these situations surgical intervention is almost always necessary.

5) Symptoms

Symptoms appear at the site where the tendon attaches to bone. A dull, achy pain is the main complaint of tendonitis sufferers, which intensifies to a sharp, excruciating pain upon activity. Specific pain occurs over the tendon and compression at this area also intensifies the pain. Tenderness and swelling may also be present accompanied by a tense, tight muscle. Some patients report grating and creaking sounds as the tendon is moved upon physical examination. The affected region may be warm and red. If there is a rupture, a gap may be felt in the tendon continuity. Tingling and numbness are not so specific for tenderness, but may occur if a nerve compression syndrome exists simultaneously.

6) Diagnosis

One should not always assume that any ache above a tendon is tendonitis. Visit a physician and/or specialist for a correct diagnosis. Tendonitis diagnosis is based on a complete physical examination, patient history taking, and relations to symptoms and signs, though medical tests such as X-rays, ultrasound and MRI may be required for differential diagnosis. A differential diagnosis is a medical condition which has the same symptoms and signs as those of tendonitis, but is a different condition altogether. In any region differential diagnosis has to be done to eliminate the likes of fractures, ligament tears, joint inflammation and/or infection, bursitis and nerve compression syndromes. These conditions can be sources of pain, tenderness, swelling, redness and numbness. Blood works such as FBP, CRP and ESR are almost always mandatory, though not for tendonitis diagnosis, but again for differential diagnosis. Tendonitis diagnosis should state what type of tendonitis it is - examples are posterior tibialis tendonitis, patellar tendonitis, rotator cuff, and tennis elbow. These are but a few. Once the correct diagnosis of tendonitis is made, the correct treatment plan is initiated.

7) How to alleviate tendonitis

Some types of tendonitis last for a few days whereas others proceed to become chronic. In most patients, chronic tendonitis, a chronic pain, is a constant nag, which many would do anything to get rid of. Tendonitis can be alleviated by using home remedies, through physiotherapy, and in severe cases- surgery.

1) The first step is to determine whether or not you have tendonitis. If you have chronic pain over a tendon that increases

when the tendon in question is stretched, it is likely that you have tendonitis.

2) The second step is to find the offending activity. This has to be something that you repeat over and over again, maybe even on a daily basis such as typing or playing tennis. Halt the activity that is in high suspicion to be the culprit. Rest for a couple of days before recommencing the activity, which may even take months before one can go back to completely doing the activity as before.

3) Apply ice to the area. This helps reduce swelling and pain. Remember not to apply ice directly to the skin. A warm bath can be used instead; however, it does not reduce inflammation, but can reduce pain. Elevating the limb at this stage is also helpful.

4) Immobilize the affected area by a brace or sling. This puts off weight at the injured site thereby reducing pain.

5) Over-the-counter pain medicines come in handy. Ibuprofen is a potent anti-inflammatory drug and is quite effective at relieving pain. If the pain is so severe that NSAIDs are ineffective to stop pain, consult your doctor.

Minimally invasive treatment methods can be introduced at this point. These are performed by your doctor.

1) Local injections such as corticosteroids, anaesthetic agents, and autologous blood can be injected at the affected tendon insertion site. These provide long-term pain relief in comparison to over-the-counter medicines. However, they do not cure tendonitis.

2) Introduce a physiotherapist to monitor and assist you with exercise routines, stretches and especially eccentric muscle stretches. A physiotherapist can also provide other alternative pain relief therapies such as laser, ultrasound and massage.

If all else fails to relieve pain in 3 months and/or when the condition is worsening, consider surgery. Surgery involves removing the inflamed tendon tissues, any calcifications, and may even require detaching and reattaching a tendon at its insertion site.

Of importance is prevention of a relapse and/or flare-up by a gradual return to daily activities and maintaining full range of motion by physical therapy. Remember to warm up before every exercise and to keep muscles warm. Too cold a muscle has a tendency to injure easily. In case you feel pain with any stretch or exercise, discontinue its proceeding.

8) Lifestyle adjustments

Lifestyle changes will help make one comfortable. These include not using the affected limb to work, for instance to carry heavy loads. Finding a temporary assistant to do chores may be of benefit. Maintain a healthy lifestyle- one which is stress-free to stay in sync physically, mentally and emotionally. Diet change may be a plus. Steer clear of sugar, alcohol, and coffee; these aggravate nerve agitation and stress. Take antioxidant remedies containing quercetin and bromelain; these help reduce swelling, as they are anti-inflammatory and neutralize metabolic wastes. A berry rich diet with dark-green and orange vegetables is helpful in damaged tissue healing. The best diet will consist of vegetables, fruits, essential oils, proteins, antioxidants, and less amounts of saturated fats and simple sugars. The use of ginger, turmeric, fish oil, bromelain, and Boswellia has also been recommended because of their naturally existing anti-inflammatory properties. Supplements that contain amino acids *glycine*, *proline* and *lysine* might help. *Glucosamine* and *chondroitine sulphate* help build proteoglycans, which are constituents of tendon extracellular matrix. Their use has been shown to be effective in joint arthritis, in particular osteoarthritis. According to online tendonitis groups, sufferers who used these medications reported to have noticed no improvement.

Tips

Develop happiness within yourself. Surround yourself with happy people; it's contagious! Do not pay attention to trivial issues and steer yourself away from stress. Nothing worsens damage than stress. Meditating for as little as 10 minutes in a day can be of benefit. Happiness, at times, depends on your self-esteem; be your own number one fan and feel good about yourself. Like any other person, problems do exist, but time passes. Recognize what you can control and what you cannot. One thing, however, is for certain; nothing is permanent. Be grateful of your blessings and appreciate them.

Chapter 3) Tendonitis of the upper limb

1) What constitutes the upper limb

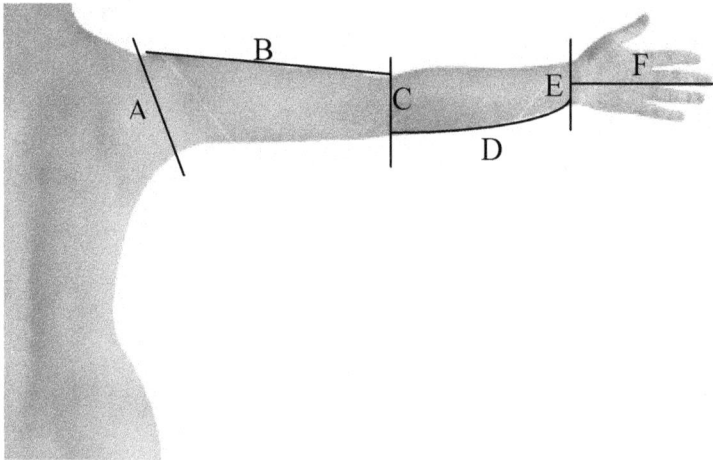

A- Shoulder joint
B- Arm or brachium
C- Elbow joint
D- Forearm or antibrachium
E- Wrist joint
F- Hand

The human body is made up of a skeleton, which can be defined as the main supporting anatomy of the organism. For vertebrates, including humans, we talk of an endoskeleton. The endoskeleton comprises each and every bone of the body to which muscles, tendons, and ligaments attach, transmitting forces for locomotion and function. The skeleton is further divided into axial skeleton, the one that forms the longitudinal axis and is made up of 80 bones in which the skull, throat, rib cage, and vertebral column are named. The axial skeleton is the weight-bearing fortress about which all the body's weight rests. The appendicular skeleton attaches to the axial one, and consists of 126 bones where the main parts constitute of the arm, forearm, hands, fingers, pelvis, thighs, legs, feet, and toes. The appendicular skeleton is per se the most mobile part of the body, consisting of two upper limbs and two lower limbs to make four appendages. In total we have 206 bones in our bodies, though individual variations can exist where extra bones are present, e.g. an extra rib.

The upper limb, also known as the upper extremity, is what is referred to by most people as the arm. It is made up of the body part from the shoulder to the hand and fingers. This portion is further divided anatomically into segments as shown in the picture on the previous page: the shoulder, arm, elbow, forearm, wrist, hand and fingers. The upper limb functions to open doors, write a book, carry things, make that swing when playing tennis, and do the crawl on a fun, sunny pool day. Any injury to the aforementioned regions can greatly compromise function.

The upper limb's segments consist of vital structures organized in such a way that function is maximized. The skin, muscles, blood vessels, nerves, and bones function hand in hand to achieve this. Each region, as far as tendonitis is concerned, has its own peculiar anatomy and muscle positioning, which makes it vulnerable or resistant to the development of tendonitis. This is covered in the following subtopics.

2) The shoulder

The shoulder is the upper limb part that allows the most movement and functions to hold the arm to the body. It allows *flexion*, when you raise your hand up as if you want a teacher to pick you to answer a question; *extension*, when you position your hand behind you with a straight elbow; *circumduction* by moving your hand on your side in circles; *abduction*, pushing your upper limb away from your body; *adduction*, moving your upper limb close to your body; *external rotation*, as in moving the back of your hand to touch your back; and *internal rotation*, touching the back of your head with your hand. All these movements allow your upper limb to respond in any direction as required by you during voluntary activity.

voluntary activity.

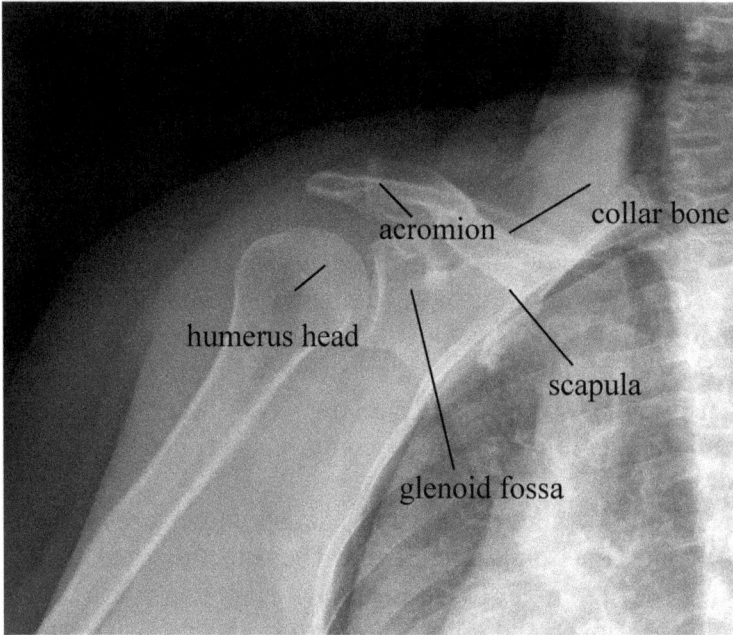

The shoulder joint is made up of an articulation of three bones: the *humerus*, which is the bone located from the shoulder to the elbow, the *scapula,* which is the winging bone at the top of your back, and the collar bone or *clavicle*. The scapula has protrusions that participate at the shoulder articulation, the cupped surface of the *glenoid fossa*. The glenoid fossa and the humerus are like a mortar and pestle rest to form a *ball-and-socket* joint. The glenoid fossa is somewhat shallow in comparison to the hip joint, and contributes to the joint stability. At this shoulder are muscles that cover the bones in cushion. The *supraspinatus, teres minor, subscapularis* and *infraspinatus* muscles are named. This sounds like medical gibberish, but they are of importance in shoulder tendonitis. These muscles are collectively called the *rotator cuff* muscles because of their arrangement around the shoulder and function; they are responsible for rotating the shoulder joint and encircle the shoulder, thus stabilizing it. The rotator cuff tendons pass under a bony prominence called the *acromion* at the top of the shoulder. A bony spur may narrow the space underneath the acromion, resulting in the impingement of the tendons at this site. With repetitive movement, the impinged tendons become inflamed and painful, resulting in tendonitis. Severe rotator cuff tendon injury may occur, resulting in a partial or a complete tendon tear. Partial results in sparing of the tendons' attachment to bone whereas complete detaches the tendon totally from its attachment site.

3) Rotator cuff tendonitis

Rotator cuff tendonitis is known by so many names: *swimmer's shoulder, pitcher's shoulder, tennis shoulder, shoulder impingement syndrome, shoulder overuse syndrome* and *tendonitis-rotator cuff*, all having the same clinical picture, same causes and same treatment plans because they are all but one disease condition. In 2000, in the U.S. about $7 billion was used in health care costs for treatment of shoulder pain. Over 33% of top swimmers experience shoulder pain, which prevents them from training; this, however, does not mean only swimmers suffer from rotator cuff tendonitis. Shoulder tendonitis is a very common cause of shoulder pain and stiffness in many individuals with a peak in those aged 40 years and beyond. Other causes such as arthritis, *bursitis* and bicipital tendonitis are also shoulder pain contributors. The *bicipital tendon* is the bicep muscle tendon which holds the humerus within the shoulder socket. Both the rotator cuff muscle tendons and the bicipital tendon can become inflamed and painful on movement, resulting in tendonitis. Between the rotator cuff tendons and the bone at the top of the shoulder, the acromion is a *bursa*, a fluid-filled sac that functions as a lubricant as the tendon moves against the bone. Inflammation of this bursa can too cause pain and stiffness at the shoulder joint.

a) Causes
Shoulder tendonitis results from sporting activities and/or professions that require repetitive shoulder use such as

swimming, baseball, tennis and golf. Factors like poor sporting technique and wrong choice of equipment can contribute to its development. Anyone can develop shoulder tendonitis, but certain factors enhance its occurrence:

a) Age - 40 years and over are susceptible to tendonitis because tendons generally degenerate with age.

b) Frequent overhead position or throwing in sporting activities and certain jobs.

c) A direct hit or bump to the shoulder and/or falling on an outstretched hand can result in acute tendonitis.

d) Other disease processes at the shoulder can result in shoulder pain and stiffness symptoms. These include arthritis of any kind e.g. rheumatoid arthritis, osteoarthritis or gout arthritis and/or infection.

One has to differentiate general shoulder tendonitis from the rotator cuff *impingement syndrome*. The position of the rotator cuff makes it vulnerable to impingement when the space between the acromion and the tendon is narrowed - see *the picture below*. This impingement causes pain and is the main mechanism by which the supraspinatus muscle gets compressed, resulting in *supraspinatus tendonitis*. 6 out of 10 causes of shoulder pain are associated with supraspinatus tendonitis.

The impingement syndrome may occur when one keeps the arm in the same position for a long time, e.g. during hairstyling or compressing the shoulder on the same side during sleep each night.

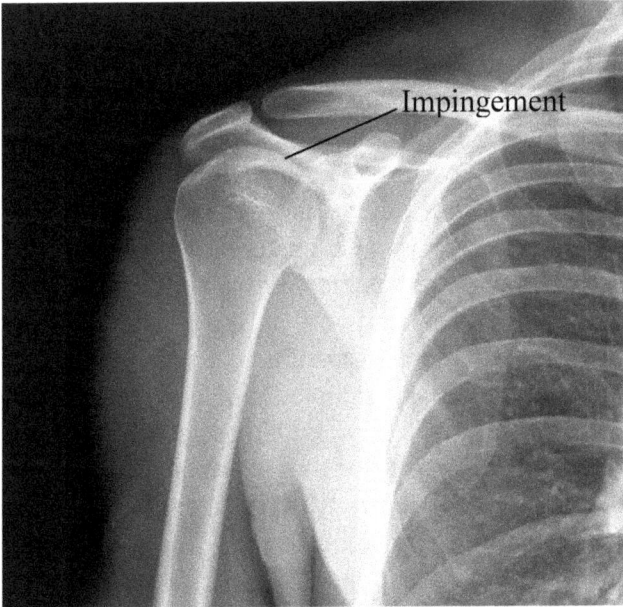

Impingement

b) When to get medical help

Most tendonitis cases disappear on their own over time, though it generally takes a few weeks to months for a complete recovery. Certain pointers need not be ignored, where one should say, "Enough is enough. I need medical consultation." Regardless of self-care at home programs, if soreness persists, intensifies, or changes course, visiting your doctor would be the right thing to do. Fever, severe swelling, heat and pain that interfere with your daily living require that you also consult with your physician. If you are taking immunosuppressive medications such as corticosteroids for asthma and/or suffer from other disease conditions like diabetes mellitus, hypertension and vascular occlusive conditions, consultation with a doctor will be of great benefit. It is, however, recommended that even if all the above does not apply to you that you visit your doctor for a correct diagnosis after which home remedies can suffice for treatment. This is so for elimination of any immediate medical pathologies, which when delayed, can be fatal to health and life e.g. septic shoulder joint.

c) Symptoms

Loss of function of the four rotator cuff muscles and/or their overuse results in their weakness, thus rendering them unable to hold the arm at the shoulder blade. Shoulder tendonitis consists of specific symptoms, which occur in varied intensities. Pain is the main complaint of most sufferers and can range from being a mild to a severe ache or sometimes is even considered to be of a sharp character that intensifies with movement. With shoulder tendonitis, pain starts mild, occurring only during activity, but as the condition progresses pain appears even at rest as a dull, constant, irritating pain. Pain may irradiate to the arm, but almost always ends before reaching the elbow. Pain that goes all the way down the upper extremity is suggestive of a nerve entrapment syndrome. If a tendon tear has occurred, a sudden severe pain occurs and a popping sound may also be heard by the patient. Rotator cuff tear pain is often experienced during the night, might even wake you up, and does not respond to painkillers. Shoulder joint movement is restricted- especially on raising the arm up and/or abduction at the joint. Weakness is yet another symptom where most patients complain of inability to lift heavy things. Warmth, swelling and redness at the shoulder joint may also exist.

d) Diagnosis

A thorough physical examination, patient history taking, symptoms and signs lead to diagnosis of the condition. A doctor checks for tenderness, restricted joint movements in certain positions, and tests for nerve function. Imaging tests and blood work are almost always done for diagnosis and differential diagnosis. X-rays may reveal impinging bony spurs, tendon calcifications and any other bone disease states. Ultrasound often reveals tendon tears if they are present and is a good eliminator of bursitis as an inflamed bursa is clearly visualized by ultrasonography. MRI is a more informative test, which can reveal soft tissue associations up to blood vessels. Specialized joint imaging like arthrography and contrast imaging may be ordered by your doctor.

e) Treatment

Swimmer's shoulder treatment consists of conservative non-surgical methods and surgical treatment options, where 78% of all rotator cuff tendonitis treated by conservative treatment were a success, and 75% of all those involved surgery. 7 stages of effective rehabilitation for this condition are essential.

Stage 1: Pain relief

As with any soft tissue injury, treatment of tendonitis involves relieving pain by the RICE method and anti-inflammatory medications such as naproxen and ibuprofen. Restricting the movement that resulted in the swimmer's shoulder in the first place is required, though to some extent movement of the joint should be maintained. A sling and/or tap for immobilization might also provide pain relief. Other methods used in stage 1 include acupuncture and massage and corticosteroid injections.

Stage 2: Achieving full range of movement (FROM)

Inflamed tendons and bursa settle if protected from further injury. Stage 1 is directed to this accord; however, healing on its own is not adequate as the injury heals with scar tissue. It is necessary to stretch these tissues to attain full range of motion. This is done by exercise, but better still by a physiotherapist. If the scar heals with no restoration of length by stretch, it contracts, forming a frozen shoulder. It is therefore important to initiate early exercise to allow full range of motion with which yields a good functional outcome.

Stage 3: Scapula control restoration

The arm is attached strongly to the chest wall by the shoulder blade (scapula). For a normal function the shoulder blade and shoulder movement are smooth, what is known as the *scapula-humeral rhythm*. A medical condition like shoulder impingement can disturb the normal scapula-humeral rhythm. Exercises and manipulations by your physiotherapist will help rehabilitate this too for a thorough effort to return a shoulder tendonitis to its full before injury function.

Stage 4: Neck and thoracic function evaluation and restoration

The body has been built in such a way that every organ or system works together with other organ systems - the shoulder is no exception. It requires the participation of the neck and thorax for complete normal function. Poor postures and pain in the neck may be referred to the shoulder. During shoulder rehabilitation it is important that your physiotherapist also evaluates the neck and scapula-thoracic joint, restoring their function by exercise if so required.

Stage 5: Rotator cuff rehabilitation

Rotator cuff muscles are the main shoulder joint function solicitors. These muscles maintain the humeral head in the glenoid fossa at rest and during function to prevent sublaxations and dislocations. Your physiotherapist will show you good exercises for strengthening the rotator cuff as by load and position. Swimmer's shoulder rehabilitation requires this muscle group to be corrected to their original strength after which stage 6 follows.

Stage 6: Function restoration

After attaining stage 5, stage 6 smoothens function by speed and power. This is done also by exercise and may require a personal trainer to reveal your sporting or work techniques to correct any biomechanical contributing factors for prevention of recurrences, also to choose the correct equipment at this stage.

Stage 7: Back to sport/work

This stage has a rehabilitated fully functioning sufferer back to the sport they love. An individual who swims should be well knowledgeable at this stage about swimmer's shoulder, its treatment and above all prevention so as to avoid relapses, at the same time maintaining speed, power and stamina. In short it is returning to be completely your old self.

Surgery

When conservative treatment measures fail to provide relief, surgical treatment is opted for. The main goal for surgery is to create more space under the acromion for the tendons. This can be achieved by removing part of the acromion, what is called *acromioplasty*, and at times removing part of the inflamed bursa. Acromioplasty can be done using keyhole techniques of arthroscopy and/or open technique surgery. Arthroscopy involves two or three puncture wounds in the shoulder where a fiber-optic scope connected to a display screen is introduced. Small instruments can be introduced into the shoulder, visualizing them on the screen to allow debridement and excision of the bone to be done. With this technique other disease states can be simultaneously treated such as joint arthritis or bicipital tendonitis. Open surgery means a surgeon makes a small incision over the shoulder- enough to visualize and carry out the procedure of the tendon and bone directly. After surgery, immobilization in a sling is done for a short period of time, after which rehabilitation by exercise is commenced. Usually it takes about 2-4 months for a complete recovery; however, other patients take as long as 1 year. Rarely do surgical complications occur, but involve infection, bleeding, stiffness and other conditions associated with anesthesia.

f) Prognosis
Many sufferers do recover completely by using a combination of medications, physiotherapy, steroid injections and other intermediate pain relief methods, though it takes weeks to several months. Those with tendon tears often require surgery, but their outcome is satisfactory and depends on factors like age, extent of tear and function before injury.

g) Tips

Do not procrastinate; take care of your tendonitis now, or it will unforgivingly abuse you for a longer time. Keep in mind that tendonitis is a short-term inflammation of the tendon. This can easily be treated, unlike tendinosis, a chronic crisis, which is a pain to heal. The subtle difference is lost for most people without medical knowledge. This book aims to simplify everything for your sake.

4) The arm

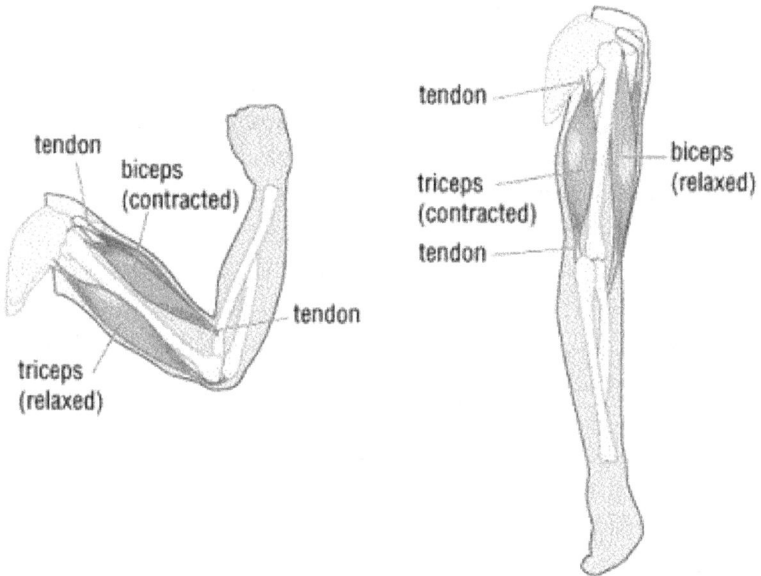

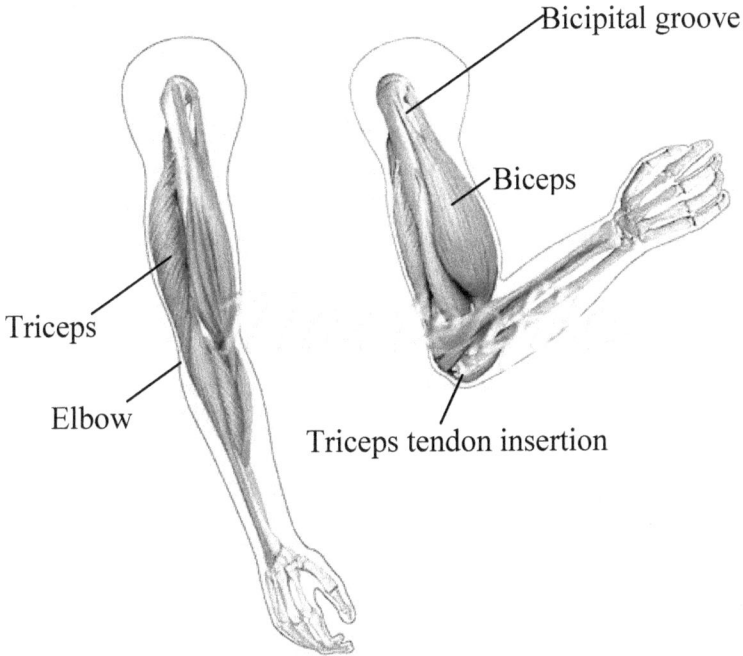

Bicipital groove

Biceps

Triceps

Elbow

Triceps tendon insertion

The arm is the region between the shoulder and the elbow. It consists of the humerus, muscles, nerves, vessels and fascia. The muscles of the arm are made up of two antagonistic groups, the *elbow flexors* and *extensors*. The term antagonist means that these muscles work as opposites - if one bends the elbow, the other straightens. The muscle group that bends the elbow consists of the *biceps, coracobrachialis* and *brachialis* muscles, whereas the extensor group has *the triceps muscle*. The biceps muscle is called "bi-" because it has two heads originating both from the scapula though at different sites. The long or lateral head starts from the top of the glenoid fossa and descends into the bicipital groove. The short head originates from the coracoid process together with the coracobrachialis muscle. The coracoids process is a bony protrusion of the scapula above the shoulder joint. These two tendons, the long head and the short, give way to two muscle bellies that unite to form the bulk of the biceps muscle. The insertion of the biceps muscle is at the *radius,* a forearm bone. The triceps is called "tri-" because it has three heads arranged in two planes. The long or lateral heads are superficially located whereas the medial head is deeper. Repetitive strain and stress of the arm result in tendonitis, in its two variants, the acute and chronic forms. The two muscles most often affected in arm tendonitis are the biceps and triceps.

5) Bicipital tendonitis

The *bicipital groove* is a furrow in the humeral bone on its top front side. At this area the long head tendon of the biceps muscle passes through as it comes from its origin point at the scapula. With each muscle contraction this tendon slides over the groove. The long head tendon of the biceps muscle is invested in a synovial sheath, a membrane which produces synovial fluid to reduce friction between the tendon and the groove. With repetitive motion and overuse, especially in overhead movements, the tendon with its synovial sheath can get irritated, inflamed and degenerate, leading to *bicipital tendonitis* and/or *bicipital tenosynovitis* if the sheath is affected. Bicipital tendonitis, tendinitis, tendinopathy or tendinosis can be described as pain in the biceps tendon accompanied by tenderness. All of those terms are used interchangeably to mean the same thing. Due to the location of the bicipital groove, which is the area more painful to compress in bicipital tendonitis, its close proximity to the shoulder makes it the most misdiagnosed musculoskeletal condition since it is confused with rotator cuff. This could explain why rotator cuff tendonitis is very frequent in comparison to many other tendonitis types. In most cases they do occur simultaneously. As the biceps tendonitis progresses, it thickens together with its synovial sheath to form a *"Popeye"* bulge which is palpable during examination.

a) Causes

Bicipital tendinopathy is caused by repetitive overhead arm overuse in activities like sport and certain jobs. Tennis, swimming, baseball and household work like painting and shoveling can be causative factors. Associated pathologies can also contribute to its development, these include shoulder girdle muscle imbalance, calcifications of the tendon, poor posture, direct trauma, impingement syndrome, chronic shoulder instability, arthritis and more.

b) Symptoms

Pain is located on the front top surface of the arm over where the bicipital groove is located. This pain is worsened by activities requiring bending the elbow or shoulder rotation and can radiate down to the elbow or up in the shoulder. Early fatigue of the biceps muscle has been reported. Swelling, warmth and tenderness can be located during physical examination. Pain is of moderate to severe intensity occurring anytime, but mostly during activity. Night pain is not uncommon.

c) Diagnosis

X-rays, CT-scans, MRI and blood works are done for differential diagnosis, but physical examination and complete patient history taking is the mainstay for bicipital tendonitis diagnosis.

d) Treatment

Treatment options always start with conservative measures, although if a tear is obvious by, let's say, MRI, surgery is the first option. RICE method should be followed and taking of NSAIDs to reduce inflammation and pain. Cortisone injections are effective anti-inflammatory medicines. They do temporarily relieve pain, but myth has it that cortisone injections cure tendonitis. This is not true because once the cortisone effects wear off, the tendonitis symptoms will resurface as before. Stretching and strengthening exercises will restore FROM and strengthen shoulder function.

When several weeks pass with no relief from conservative measures or if the condition worsens, surgery should be considered. In bicipital tendonitis, arthroscopy is usually the performed procedure. Any tears can be repaired. In some cases a procedure called *tenodesis* is done. In this operation the damaged tendon section is excised, with reattachment of the remaining tendon to the humerus. In severe cases, when a surgeon cannot repair the tendon and/or *tenodes*, a *tenotomy* is performed. This is complete resection of the biceps tendon from its attachment site at the top of the glenoid fossa.

Surgery complications are rare, but if they occur are usually associated with infection, bleeding and problems associated with anesthesia. Recovery is often a success in most operated cases, though post surgery rehabilitation is required and should be followed depending on your doctor's orders. A temporary sling or brace is applied for immobilization in the first few days to allow tendon healing to occur. Once the post-op soreness disappears full rehabilitation is commenced, starting with stretches then over to strengthening exercises. Speed and power is the target of the last rehabilitation stage with return to work and/or sport.

e) Tips

Carrying your toddler, like any parent, is a bonding activity, which can never be avoided. Prevent pain by using a baby carrier in front or the back. If you really have to carry your baby, avoid sitting your child on one arm but use both hands, one supporting the other.

6) Triceps tendonitis

Triceps tendonitis is inflammation of the triceps muscle. This is actually a misnomer because most overuse injuries to any tendon are called tendinopathies, so the actual name should be triceps tendinopathy. However, triceps tendonitis, triceps tendinosis and *triceps tendinopathy* are all used to mean the same condition. The triceps muscle is the bulk of muscle you feel above the elbow, but at the back of the arm. The triceps muscle originates from the shoulder blade and humerus, inserting into the ulna- the forearm bone you feel as a pointed structure at the back of the elbow. Contracting the triceps muscle transmits force through the triceps tendon to straighten the elbow; therefore, its function is to straighten the elbow joint and is called an *elbow extensor muscle*. Repetitive use and/or overstrain of the triceps tendon, like many body tendons results in its inflammation and degeneration causing pain and restricted movement. This is often a chronic condition occurring over time and/or may be acute when a high force going through the triceps tendon beyond what it can withstand is exerted.

a) Causes
Triceps tendonitis usually occurs by repetitive stress injuries of pushing activities or straightening the elbow against resistance for a long time such as pushups and bench presses. Acute form arises from lifting heavy things like weightlifting in the gym beyond your stamina. There are some predisposing factors to triceps tendinopathy, including obesity, elbow joint stiffness, inadequate warm-up before exercising, muscle weakness, inappropriate training techniques and triceps muscle tightness.

b) Symptoms
Pain in the back of the elbow that occurs during activities requiring strong triceps muscle contractions such as boxing or dips is characteristic. The pain may be accompanied by elbow stiffness that limits joint mobility. As the condition progresses, the pain may become sharp, appearing even at rest. Swelling, redness and tenderness at the back of the elbow are possible.

c) Diagnosis
Physical, subjective, and objective elbow examination by a doctor or physiotherapist, in combination with life history, symptoms and signs, is often adequate for a diagnosis. Further medical investigations as always are done, X-rays, CT-scan and/or MRI are important for differential diagnosis. Blood works such as CRP, FBP and ESR are recommended.

d) Treatment

Like any other tendonitis, depending on condition extent, patient's health and other factors involved, resting, ice, compression and elevation, NSAIDs for pain relief, sling and/or splinting the elbow temporarily in a brace are the main home treatment modalities. Massage, acupuncture, corticosteroid injections, ABI and PRP can also be used for pain relief. Ultrasound and shockwave therapies are also methods that can be implemented. Physiotherapy stretches and exercises are the main rehabilitation processes.

e) Prognosis

With appropriate medication, rehabilitation and physiotherapy, most patients heal completely in a number of weeks, though that may extend to several months.

7) The elbow

The elbow is the joint between the arm and the forearm. It is a pivot point for flexion and extension of the upper limb, and thus allows the main function of the upper extremity to be fulfilled. Unlike the shoulder joint, which is a ball and socket, the elbow is a hinge joint allowing movement in only two planes, that is flexion and extension. The elbow joint is formed by three bones articulating together, the humerus, *radius* and *ulna*. These bones are invested in a *joint capsule* formed by ligaments, which stabilize the joint. The joint capsule is lined by a *synovial membrane,* which produces *synovial fluid* for friction-free joint mobility, as this fluid acts as a lubricant. Ligaments connect bone to bone, and are of importance to prevent overriding of the articulation into a subluxation and/or a dislocation. Besides ligaments, the elbow joint is further stabilized by muscles, which act around and cushion the joint. Muscles are covered by a sheath called a *fascia,* which is in itself a collagen-formed substance. Blood vessels and nerves run through the joint from the shoulder on their way to supply the lower-lying structures of the forearm, wrist and hand.

Repetitive stress of overuse on any part of the body where tendons are located almost always results in tendonitis over time; the elbow is not spared by this rule. At the elbow, the forearm muscle tendons are attached on the epicondyles of the humerus. *Epicondyles* are bony prominences formed by the knobbed distal segment of the humerus. If you half bend your elbow and palpate on your elbow sides you can feel bone protrusions sticking out, these are the epicondyles. The epicondyle on the inside of the elbow surface is called the medial or inner epicondyle, whereas the one outer is termed the lateral or outer epicondyle. Anywhere on the human body where *lateral* and *medial* terms are used mean far from the centre of the body and near to the centre, respectively. At these epicondyles are attached tendons of forearm flexor and extensor muscle groups.

Forearm flexor muscle tendons originate from a single *origin* point, the medial epicondyle where repetitive micro-injury on these tendons can cause *medial epicondylitis*, which is also known as *golfer's elbow*. Epicondylitis per se, as some specialists call it, is a myth, since upon direct open view of the epicondyles the muscle tendons are seen to appear as if they are ligaments and they do not exhibit the gliding characteristics of true tendons. However you look at it, in this context these terms still apply since their use is worldwide. On the lateral epicondyle is attached the forearm extensor muscle tendon. Their injury results in *lateral or outer epicondylitis*, which is also known as *tennis elbow*.

Epicondylitis is a medical condition affecting age ranges between 30-60 years, with a male dominance, though research has proven this to be statistically insignificant. Pain and tenderness at the elbow are the main symptoms of epicondylitis, though many other disease states such as arthritis, *olecranon bursitis*, triceps tendonitis, infection and nerve compression syndrome also may have these signs. This points out that a proper diagnosis by a physician is required for the correct diagnosis to be made. However, after diagnosis one can completely treat epicondylitis at home by following physiotherapy exercises and stretches, plus home remedies and/or natural treatment modalities.

8) Tennis elbow

Tennis elbow or lateral epicondylitis is inflammation and degeneration of the extensor tendon attachment at the lateral epicondyle, occurring in 5% of all cases of tennis players. It is a slow and gradual tendon condition, which has episodic flare-ups. Tennis elbow arises due to activities that cause overstrain on the lateral epicondyle tendon such as sport and certain jobs. Tennis, basketball, baseball, javelin, especially using poor technique, cause tennis elbow. This does not mean, however, that only poor technique in sport causes tennis elbow; predisposing factors too, like age and concomitant diseases of inflexibility and joint stiffness cause tennis elbow. It is very important for sport lovers to understand the chance of tennis elbow development and how to protect oneself. In tennis, playing lightweight rackets, a rough court, one-handed backstrokes, hitting the ball late and biomechanically unstable positions increase the probability of tennis elbow.

Symptoms of tennis elbow start gradually as a dull ache that appears only during activity on the outer surface of the elbow. With progression it sharpens, occurring even at rest. Tenderness at the lateral epicondyle is typical with swelling and at times warmth. Radial nerve compression at the elbow results in tennis elbow-like symptoms, which make it difficult to make correct diagnoses. Radial nerve compression, however, has tingling and the pain radiates towards the wrist. Physical examination by a doctor using the see, feel, and move principle proposed by Apleys is adequate. Specific maneuvers are done to substantiate the disease condition; the chair lifting test can be done. With a straight elbow, a patient lifts the back of a chair using three fingers - the thumb, index and middle fingers. Severe pain at the outer elbow is a positive test. Differential diagnosis is required, first from radial nerve compression where nerve condition tests are helpful. A *Tinel sign* is performed by tapping over the skin lying above the nerve with a finger. If a tingling sensation or numbness appears or worsens, the test is said to be positive.

Treatment begins with modifying sport playing choices, things like racket selection - racket quality of size, grip, weight and string tension. 11 ounces is the recommended weight that has shock-absorbing capacity. Looser strings are thought to reduce force exerted on the tendon by delaying transferred shock to the forearm from the ball impact through stretch. A grip size comfortable to your hand size is recommended. Tennis ball size and weight also matters. A wet ball is heavy and hence requires an increased force effort by each swing. The speed in which a ball bounces is also taken into account and depends on the surface on which it lands. A hard court is very brutal to the elbow and clay is by many the recommended surface. Other court surfaces exist like grass and their effect is unpredictable, but then again in tennis, elbow extensor tendon overuse is the enemy.

Cortisone shots at the tender tendon site are effective in a great number of patients, though their relief is temporary. Botox injection is currently under research as Botox, a botulism toxin, temporarily paralyses muscles, allowing tendons to rest and heal. RICE method, splinting, NSAIDs and exercises are still by far the best home initial tendon injury therapy, though shockwave and ultrasound therapies are also used by physiotherapists. Natural managements using diet and supplements can be implemented and at times are combined with needle or laser acupuncture. Surgery is indicated in prolonged, non-settling tendonitis and involves debridement and/or detachment and reattachment of the inflamed tendon. This too can be done by open surgery and/or keyhole techniques. Whichever way a sufferer opts to have their tennis elbow treated, the good news is that if all principles are followed, 95% of all non-surgically treated cases are shown to successfully heal and 80-90% of those treated by using surgery.

Tips

Everyday things like washing your car, taking a shower, and brushing teeth can be improved by a few lifestyle changes. First advice is to listen to your body. Do not be a macho; if any activity gives you the slightest feeling of pain, do not ignore it. Avoid the task and implement pain and inflammation relief protocols. The 2 + 2 = 5 rule works where you do both physiotherapy and take NSAIDs to allow for synergy. Icing by using the RICE method is still appropriate. A tip in winter is to use snow, or in summer, crush the ice, since cold water and frozen bottles do not emit cold enough. Also, icing while sitting can result in less motivation; use neoprene wrap with a cold pack inside. It allows you to walk around while icing. For tennis players, change your serve motion by concentrating on a forward, not upward, movement and change strings to x-1 at tension, no more than 60. Technical glitches in your playing may include gripping the racquet too tightly, not completely following through with a swing, and missing the center of the racquet face. Check racquetball-lessons.com for smooth, effortless, efficient playing techniques.

9) Golfer's elbow

Golfer's elbow contrary to its name does not only occur in golf players, but to anyone, especially those above 40 years of age with reduced tendon collagen production and function. Golfer's elbow, also known as medial epicondylitis, a medical condition where there is pain and tenderness on the bony prominence on the inside of the elbow. It occurs less frequently than tennis elbow, but is pathophysiologically an overuse tendon injury as a tennis elbow and/or any other tendonitis. Golfer's elbow occurs as an acute injury with direct trauma to the tendon, an example being bumping the elbow on a hard surface, or it can have a slow gradual repeated micro-trauma, which accumulates over time to result in medial epicondylitis symptoms at some point. Nirschl proposed 4 stages of epicondylar tendinosis after years of research in tendinopathies. These stages apply to both tennis and golfer's elbow.

Stage1 - consists of tendon inflammation.

Stage 2 - tendon tissues are altered. Here, collagen-producing cells make a less strong collagen type, type III instead of type I. This results in tendon tissue of a reduced tensile strength, rendering it weak and open to repeated stress injuries.

Stage 3 - the changed tissue character leads to tendon failure.

Stage 4 - stages 2 and 3 are repeated over and over. As the tendon gets micro-trauma it attempts to repair itself. This causes formation of a thick fibrous tissue within the tendon, altering its initial structure. In a correct environment calcifications also occur.

10-20% of all diagnosed epicondylitis constitute of gofer's elbow, symptoms of which mimic tennis elbow - the only difference being it occurs on the opposite side of the elbow. Pain and tenderness occurring on the medial elbow surface radiating to the medial forearm towards the wrist is typical. Warmth and swelling may also be present. Differential diagnosis is important, and is against other elbow medical states such as ulnar nerve compression in its groove behind the medial epicondyle. Ulnar nerve entrapment, called the cubital nerve syndrome, results in tingling and paraesthesia on the medial forearm and wrist, the small and ring fingers. Again, Dr. Nirschl defined 3 zones of ulnar nerve differential diagnosis. The first zone is the area above the medial epicondyle; the second is the medial epicondyle itself, and third being below it. These zones show areas of possible ulnar nerve compression in patients with both golfer's and cubital nerve syndrome. Zone 3 was proven by Nirschl to be the most common site.

A doctor performs the golfer's elbow test to confirm diagnosis. In this test, a patient's elbow is in a straight position with the palm facing up. The doctor puts a thumb on the medial epicondyle, and with the other hand flexes the elbow, rotating the forearm to face the palm down with simultaneous flexion of the wrist and fingers towards them. Pain running along the medial forearm marks a positive test.

After, a correct diagnosis treatment is initiated. Refer to treatment scheme under tennis elbow, for it is the same with a difference on surgical intervention. A tendon debridement and reattachment procedure can be done, but at the medial epicondyle, within the same procedure. The ulnar nerve repositioning is done if cubital nerve syndrome is also present.

Tips

Typing is among the repetitive motions that cause golfer's elbow. Improve your condition by using a joy-stick type mouse or Quill. You can also use an ergonomic keyboard while wearing a golfer's brace. The best option, if available, is to use speech writing software. These, unfortunately, have their own user issues, like the requirement of teaching the software to understand you.

10) The Forearm

The part between the wrist and the elbow is called the forearm, also known as the *antibrachium*. The antibrachium has two bones, the radius and the ulna, which form a joint at either end. The *proximal radioulnar joint* allows for the radius to revolve around the ulna during supination. The distal radioulnar joint is a short distance from the wrist. Between the radius and the ulna is the *interosseus membrane.* Muscles of the forearm are separated into two groups by a fascial compartment, flexors and extensors. The anterior group has superficial, intermediate and deep layers, though all function to flex the wrist and the fingers. The flexors are innervated by the median nerve, which runs along the anterior forearm muscle compartment. All the flexors have the same origin point, which is the medial epicondyle, where inflammation and overuse will cause medial epicondylitis. The named muscles include *flexor carpi ulnaris, palmaris longus, flexor carpi radialis and pronator teres,* etc. The posterior compartment of the forearm consists of wrist and finger extensors. They are divided into superficial and deep layers where *extensor digitorum, extensor carpi ulnaris*, *extensor carpi radialis brevis* and *longus* are examples. They start from the lateral epicondyle. Overuse and inflammation of their tendons causes tennis elbow. The posterior compartment is supplied by the radial nerve injury to which a wrist drop arises.

11) Forearm tendonitis

Tendonitis is inflammation and degeneration of the thick fibrous bands connecting muscles to bone. Forearm tendonitis constitutes inflammation of tendons of the forearm. This often occurs when people all of a sudden increase the intensity of their training and/or its frequency. Other pre-tendonitis factors can be predisposing to its occurrence, such as muscle weakness, muscle imbalance and genetic susceptibility. Forearm tendonitis affects most fitness enthusiasts and weightlifters. It can also occur from sports like tennis and/or working on the computer. One concept that most need to understand is that muscles gain bulk and strength faster than tendons such that a weight overload affects tendons differently if compared to muscles, especially in bodybuilders. So, one should not assume that tendon and muscle physique is the same when stepping up exercise routines. Tendons however are strong per unit area in comparison to muscle; it's just that they take time to reach a particular strength.

a) Symptoms

In the forearm two zones are prone to pain. These are identified as the area just below the elbow on the front of the forearm and the second zone being on the anterior of the forearm just before the wrist. Pain and tenderness in these zones are typical of forearm tendonitis and it runs along the forearm, but is localized within the forearm. The pain feels like pulling tense muscles, like a mild cramp occurring more in the morning and at night. Activity exacerbates pain such that a simple activity like raising a coffee mug to the mouth might be very painful. Swelling and redness is typical of forearm tendonitis and is more visible in fair- or light-skinned people. Differential diagnosis is always necessary in this case from fractures, *pyomyositis*, which is pus accumulation in a muscle, and muscle contusions. One medical emergency that you need to be on the lookout for is a *heart attack*. It is felt as a forearm pain originating from deep within the chest through the shoulder to the forearm and radiating to the hand and fingers. The emergency services have to be called immediately if this is encountered.

b) Diagnosis
Diagnosis is supported mainly by a thorough medical examination. Other tests, however, are ordered to substantiate the diagnosis and/or to rule out other candidate diagnosis.

c) Treatment
Signs and symptoms, the affected region, movement restrictions and pain on resisted movement constitute a positive forearm tendonitis diagnosis and treatment should be started immediately. The initial goal of treatment is to relieve pain and inflammation, ice pack massages, NSAIDs and rest are necessary. One should seek further treatment if home remedies do not work. Many other treatment substitutes exist, but are not for self-administration, including cortisone shots, ABI, shockwave therapy, etc. Many sufferers do completely recover, but after so much patience and effort.

d) Prevention
Prevention is the best cure for any condition and in forearm tendonitis, it involves changing routine techniques. For instance, bicep curls using a straight bar has high resistance and one might opt for a Z-curl bar instead. Warming up before exercise allows your body to adjust to stress before exerting heavy duty exercise plans.

12) The wrist and hand
The hand and the wrist are the most functional parts of the upper extremity without which a person cannot touch, hold, carry and/or open things. Physicians are dealing with hand and wrist disorders on a daily basis, from closed and open injuries to traumatic fractures and disease states such as arthritis. The wrist and hand,

like the gross anatomy of any body area constitutes of skin, muscles, ligaments, tendons, nerves, vessels and bones. They are divided by side to the *dorsum*, which is the back side of the hand, and the *palmer* side located at the front. The skin of the dorsal hand is thin and vascularized by lymphatic and blood vessels such that it often swells worse than the palmer side if injured. The palmer surface has a thickened skin with a lot of pores to allow a fixed adequate grip during function. The wrist has two muscle groups, which are continuous with the forearm, the flexor and extensor muscle groups, the flexors being located on the side continuous with the palm of the hand. Within the hand are intrinsic and extrinsic muscles, which play the major role of finger movement. At the wrist, the flexors and extensors form long tendons that enter the hand. These tendons are the *flexor digitorum tendons* and the *extensor digitorum*. Before they leave the wrist to enter the hand they are bound by a thick fibrous band called *retinaculi* which surrounds the wrist like a half bracelet on either side. The *flexor retinaculum* holds the flexor digitorum tendons in place and it is at this region where the median nerve entrapment syndrome often occurs, otherwise known as carpal tunnel syndrome. The flexor retinaculum is positioned about 2 centimeters from the wrist onto the palm whereas the *extensor retinaculum* is just at the wrist but at the back of the wrist.

The digitorum tendons attach to the bones of the finger, which are also called digits or phalanges, in such a way that a deep and a superficial tendon attachment exists. The deep attachment allows for bending of the proximal segment of the digit while the superficial the distal end. The distal end of a digit is the pole where the nail is located and the proximal is the opposite upward direction. The tendons are surrounded by the synovial sheath to allow easy and smooth loading during function.

A total count of 27 bones are located at the wrist and hands. The wrist is formed by the lower segment of the ulna and radius articulating with the *carpal bones*. Carpal bones are 8 arranged at the wrist in 2 rows of 4. They are continuous with the *metacarpals* and the fingers. All fingers, except the thumb, which has 2, have 3 segments. On these bones are ligaments connecting bone to bone. At the wrist the ligaments form a joint capsule, which is lined by a synovial membrane containing its synovial fluid. Fingers are also joined by ligaments at every joining segment, which form small joint capsules. These capsules are also lubricated for smooth sailing of the fingers. Blood supply at the hand and wrist is supplied by two main arteries, which descend from the parent artery, the brachial artery. These are called the ulna and radial arteries and they anastemose or join at the palmer surface and the dorsum hand to form arcs which are deep and superficial. These arcs form small tributaries to supply the whole hand. The radial, ulnar and median nerves are the ones responsible for motor and sensory innervation of this upper limb segment.

13) Wrist tendonitis

Tendons at the wrist consist of synovial sheaths, and when they get irritated and inflamed by overuse, a tenosynovitis also occurs. Tenosynovitis results in tendon enlargement as scar tissue forms in an attempt to heal by the tendon. These lumps can be large and cause wrist space compression and in the end a carpal tunnel syndrome arises. *Carpal tunnel syndrome* and wrist tendonitis/tenosynovitis are inseparable. Carpal tunnel syndrome is a median nerve compression resulting in the nerve being squashed and damaged through its passage from the wrist to the hand. All these conditions cause wrist or forearm pain, which varies from person to person in intensity and character. Wrist tendonitis pain comprises of an on-and-off character, though in some sufferers appears even at rest. A burning sensation and/or tingling may be felt in the hand. Due to scar tissue formation, movement at the wrist and fingers is restricted and stiff, and tendons lose their smooth gliding effect. Warmth at the joint or heat, swelling and redness are not uncommon.

Wrist tendonitis can be identified when an individual experiences irritation, pain, burning and tingling sensations at the wrist. Activities such as sewing, bowling, typing, catching and hitting ball are the main activities associated. People aged over 30 are the usual sufferers.

Treatment of wrist tendonitis involves general tendonitis treatment concepts.

Tips

With wrist tendonitis, daily chores can be depressing. We have some tips to help you go by. Ask your partner or family members for help to spread the bed, to load and unload the washer, and even to carry things. They understand what you are going through more than you may know. But, some chores can be made easy, like scrubbing sinks and tubs. Use lime scale sprays and scum busters available in local shops, Wal-Mart, and Tesco. They do the job for you.

Sleeping techniques may worsen wrist tendonitis. Sleep with your hand flat on a pillow and not bent it or put it in a fist, keeping them warm by Handeze gloves available on Amazon.com. The strangest thing I have encountered is that some sufferers swear by copper bracelets. Just wearing copper over the wrist has been reported to relieve pain. Is it because copper cools the wrist? This theory has no scientific explanation, but trying it may be fun.

What is the difference between wrist tendonitis and carpal tunnel?

Carpal tunnel syndrome is a common condition involving tingling and burning sensations in the hands, often felt at night. The numbness affects the thumb, index finger, middle finger and half of the ring finger. Other symptoms are thumb weakness, a feeling of pricking pins and needles, and a constant dull hand pain associated with the hand being heavy. The median nerve passes at the wrist on the anterior forearm area where it often gets compressed in its tunnel or passage. Compression can be caused by injuries to the wrist that heal with fibrous tissue; diabetes and rheumatoid arthritis are frequent accompanying disease states and 50% of pregnant women complain of its symptoms. Carpal tunnel is treated with steroid injections, splints and exercises, but with time often ends up requiring surgery to decompress the tunnel by removing the restricting components.

Tendonitis symptoms mimic those of carpal tunnel syndrome and it is no surprise that the two are often confused, though a few differences exist. Pain on the front or palm side of the wrist is more suggestive of a carpal tunnel syndrome, whereas one localized at the back of the wrist is for tendonitis. Needle and pins sensation is more in carpal tunnel syndrome. This is not true though for all cases so still it's a tricky situation since the correct diagnosis is important, because median nerve decompression surgery will not relieve tendonitis and vice versa. A nerve conduction test may be a great tool to check the nerve function; its compromise will point out carpal tunnel syndrome, though a simultaneous occurrence is still possible.

14) Hand tendonitis

When after work you feel a certain ache in your fingers that does not seem to improve or go away, this is a sign of hand tendonitis. Hand tendonitis is associated with pain and tenderness located along the tendons; sometimes patients confuse it for joint pain. Repetitive movement and work like miners and road works worsen this condition. Other diseases such as arthritis and diabetes may have such symptoms, so differentiation should be picked up on by a physician. Stiffness in joints and tenderness are also among sufferer's complaints.

Hand tendon inflammation and degeneration results in hand tendonitis. It's an overuse injury, though rarely, direct injury may cause acute hand tendonitis. Diagnosis is by physical examination, X-rays and blood work for differential diagnosis. It is of importance to mention the two main tendonitis types associated with hand tendonitis, *trigger finger* and *De Quervain's* tendonitis.

Tips

Unhooking or hooking a bra from behind can feel like rock climbing if one is suffering from hand tendonitis. A tip to prevent severe pain is to buy a bra with clasps in the front. These bras do exist but may be difficult to find; check www.barenecessities.com, eBay, and www.macys.com. If you use the ones with clasps positioned behind, fasten your bra in front and then spin the clasp around to the back. Your hair styling can also be compromised by pain occurring in prolonged hair drying. Instead, go to the salon and let someone else do it for you. Salons, however, can be expensive; you can still do this by yourself at home, try salon type dryers, check Conair HH400 Ionic salon dryer from Amazon.

Hand and foot tendonitis usually occurs in rheumatoid arthritis patients. If this is your case, you could grind garlic and mix it with warm aloe lotion. Use this mixture to massage your feet and your hands.

15) Trigger finger

Trigger finger, also called *stenosing tenosynovitis,* is marked by a finger fixing its position in a bent way. When it straightens, a snap is heard like a released gun trigger, hence the name trigger finger. It is a very painful condition associated with narrowing of space between the tendon and its synovial sheath. This causes the tendon to stiffen and become difficult to move.

Trigger finger is, by definition, a disease condition where a tendon and its synovial sheath get inflamed for a prolonged period so that a fibrous tissue scar forms. This condition is very common in diabetic patients and in those with rheumatoid arthritis.

Symptoms include stiffness of fingers, which is more present in the morning. One has to stretch fingers before use, and a popping or snapping sound can be heard as it straightens, with locking and catching of the finger in a bent position. Bumps and nodules form along the tendons due to scarring. Trigger finger affects mostly the thumb, index, middle or ring finger on the dominant hand.

This condition, however is not the same as thickening and contracture of the *palmer aponeurosis*, what is known as *Dupuytren's contracture*. Diagnosis does not require medical tests. Medical history and physical examination are adequate for a correct diagnosis.

In mild forms, treatment involves the usual, RICE method, NSAIDs and corticosteroid injections, exercises and avoiding repetitive overuse of the fingers. Most patients have been shown to respond well to corticosteroid injections. If no relief is achieved, then surgery can be performed, which is aimed at increasing the space of tendon passage on the fingers. Percutaneous trigger tendon release can be done, where under local anaesthesia, a needle is used to release the locked finger. Open surgical tendon release is done in severe cases. Complications are relapse of the condition and/or its incomplete treatment. Infection, though rare, might also occur.

Tips

Phone texting is a repetitive motion, and one might actually suffer from "texting tendonitis." For those who cannot be separated from their smartphones, and even regular phones, finger pain is an unpleasant burden, especially if you are connected to many people who are always on chat with you. The pain often appears after using the phone to reply to long messages on Whatsapp for many hours and/or playing games for long periods at a time. This pain may radiate to the forearm, elbow, and shoulders. Hand exercises are, as always, a solution, but a lot of praise has been given to hot water jets and soaking. Other changes that can be made to improve your condition are as follows:

1) Prevent repetitive stress to a single finger by often changing the typing finger.

2) Reply or write short messages.

3) Buy a huge-sized phone with large buttons. This prevents strain by making it easy to type.

4) Take breaks in between using your phone.

Other medical conditions may also be associated with texting, such as forward head posture and carpal tunnel syndrome. Because this texting problem is becoming frequent with many people getting addicted to their phones, Facebook, or Twitter, medical professionals have devised a mobile application, "Achebreak," to remind you to take breaks and exercise in between texting; see http://www.AchebreakApp.com.

16) De Quervain's tendonitis

De Quervain's tendonitis is pain and tenderness occurring at the base of the thumb. Two tendons of the thumb form a pulley system at the wrist, where if irritation and inflammation occurs, tendonitis results. De Quevain's tendonitis occurs in diabetic patients, pregnant women and those with rheumatoid arthritis, though not all. This is so because systemic diseases like rheumatoid arthritis have systemic inflammatory substances circulating in the blood. These substances initiate inflammation when a trigger factor is present, in this case repetitive overuse. Symptoms of De Quervain's consist of pain at the base of the thumb and area beside the wrist. This pain appears gradually, but sudden onset has been reported.

Gripping and squeezing worsens the pain, which may radiate to the forearm. Snapping and popping sounds are not uncommon and so is numbness around the thumb and the index finger.

The *Finkelstein tes*t is done to confirm diagnosis. In this test, a fist is made with the fingers closing over the thumb, and the wrist bending towards the little finger. This maneuver causes the passage of thumb tendons to be reduced, resulting in tendon compression, which if it is inflamed, sudden sharp pain is excited. Treatment modalities are aimed at pain relief and restoration of function. Splints of the thumb or wrist, NSAIDs, corticosteroid injections and rest do calm pain in most sufferers. Surgery, if it is required, involves creating space or room for the thumb tendons to move freely.

Tips

De Quervain's tendonitis can cause pain in daily life activities. One can reduce the extent of this pain by learning a few tips and skills. For example, holding a toothbrush can be such a stress that you may even choose to skip this daily hygiene routine; buy an electric toothbrush instead. That way, you will get to brush your teeth with comfort.

Chapter 4) Tendonitis of the lower limb

1) Constituents of the thigh

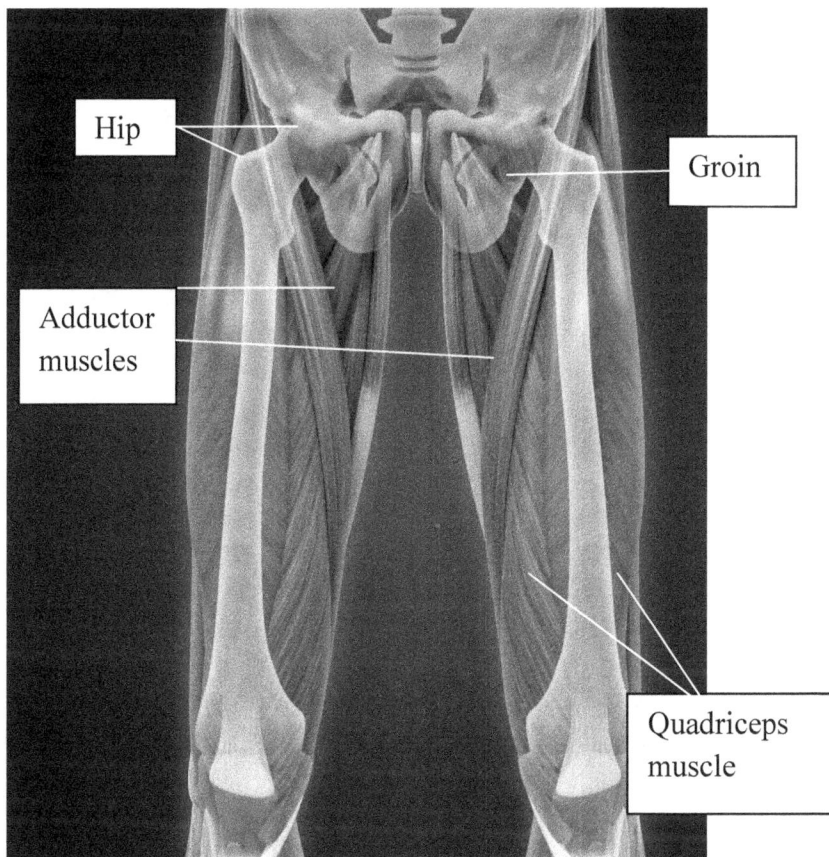

The lower limb consists of 6 major parts: the hip girdle, thigh, knee, leg, ankle and foot. Its function is to support the body during locomotion and to balance the body in space. Anatomically, these regions have specific names which are used by specialists: *coxa* (hip), *femur* (thigh bone), *genu* (knee), *crus* (leg), *sura* (calf), *talus* (ankle), and *pes or pedis* (foot). Under the foot is the plantar surface - the heel is *calx* and *hallux* means the big toe. The lower limb, if you look closely, has segments like those of the upper limb. The ankle correlates with the wrist, as it joins the tarsals, metatarsals and toes in place of carpals, metacarpals and fingers in the upper limb.

The hip joint is a ball-and-socket joint where the thigh bone's head sits in a hollow ridge on the side of the pelvis, the *acetabulum*. This shape enhances joint stability, which is re-enforced by the *labrum* and ligaments. A labrum is the rubbery half circle surrounding the hip joint, thus deepening the ball and socket even further. Ligaments crisscross around the hip joint attaching on the *intertrochanteric line* and the acetabular margins. These ligaments form a joint capsule, which fixes the head of the femur within the acetabulum, preventing subluxation and dislocation. Per se the hip joint is like the shoulder joint, a difference being that the shoulder ball and socket is shallow. Synovial fluid as a lubricant is produced within the joint capsule. Muscles overlie the joint to give an even more stable structure. The *gluteal* muscles, *iliopsoas*, *adductors* and thigh muscles do support the joint. The iliopsoas, pectineus and femoral vessels together with the femoral, obturator and sciatic nerves supply the joint.

The hip and the groin, though both are located at the junction between the pelvis and thigh, are 2 different regions. The term *groin* is used to mean the inside thigh region below the inguinal crease. Groin muscles start from the inner thigh and attach to the inner pelvis. These muscles are called adductor muscles and include the *adductor longus, adductor brevis, adductor magnus, gracilis* and *pectineus*, forming the medial compartment of the thigh. Adductor muscles function to stabilize the hip and pull the hip and thigh inward when they contract. The injury and inflammation of their tendons result in *adductor tendonitis*, which is also known as the groin pull.

When we talk of the hip, we generally mean the area at your waist that you touch when you are told to place your hands on your hips- where a bony protrusion marks the location, the *greater trochanter*. At the greater trochanter, hip rotating muscles attach and the gluteal muscle group, among others, is named. A bursa is located nearby and acts as a shock absorber for these rotator muscle tendons, the *trochanteric bursa*, inflammation of which results in *trochanteric bursitis*.

From the hip to the knee is the thigh, which is divided into 3 muscle compartments by a fascial intermuscular septa. The anterior, medial and posterior muscle groups encompass a single long bone called the femur. The medial (inner) compartment has the adductor muscles; the posterior has the knee-bending *hamstring muscle* and the leg-extending quadriceps muscle interiorly. In each compartment are nerves running between muscles to innervate their motor and sensory activity. It is also important to mention the blood supply of the femoral artery, femoral vein and lymphatic vessels, which move in the *adductor canal*. The great saphenous vein adjoins the femoral vein at the *femoral triangle* and is responsible for varicose veins in some patients.

Pain at the hip and thigh can be due to many reasons, one of which is pain radiating from a compressed nerve root at the back. This compression can occur due to lumbar degenerative joint disease (DJD) or a lumbar herniated disc. Spinal stenosis and sacroiliac joint dysfunction are also possible causes. Pain in these cases is located at the lower back, thighs, groin and moves down the leg, giving numbness and tingling sensations with or without muscle power grade reduction. Local hip joint problems, such as trochanteric bursitis, hip fracture, hip muscle strain, pelvis fracture and hip arthritis are often leading causes of hip pain, as hip and thigh muscles do also attach to the bones in this area. Their overuse can result in tendinopathies. In the following pages, hip, groin, quadriceps and hamstring tendonitis are discussed.

2) Hip tendonitis

Active individuals who participate in cycling, running, and soccer, etc. may suffer from *hip tendonitis*. This may occur as an acute muscle strain or develop over time into the chronic form. Poor activity techniques, increasing exercise training suddenly and pre-existing conditions may predispose one to hip tendonitis development. Anyone can suffer from a hip tendinopathy, but those who are active are top listed. The tendinous part of any muscle has poor blood supply, so overstressing these zones can result in degeneration. Degeneration, as we understand it, is associated with hypocellularity, a switch in collagen fiber types and formation of a scar tissue which causes the tendon to thicken. In children, the presentation is somewhat different since muscles attach to growing bones with growth plates. Any inflammation will result in apophysitis and/or tendon weakness, which results in complete pulling off of the tendon and the growth plate.

Pain is the main patient complaint in hip tendonitis. This pain should be described adequately. That is, is the pain sudden or is it developed gradually? After what activity did the pain occur, e.g. abrupt deceleration, and was the patient able to use the limb after injury? A sudden pop or snap with a localized severe pain and inability to use the limb may be suggestive of a tendon tear. Many other questions can be asked by a physician during history taking. Is the patient on any medications? Has the condition ever happened before? What aggravates or alleviates symptoms? Other possible sources of pain should be ruled out and include spinal associated diseases like disc herniation, gynecological symptoms may also elicit hip pain, but are usually associated with other complaints like amenorrhea, menstrual irregularities and per vaginal discharge. Abdominal cramps may radiate to the hip, but include nausea, vomiting, stool pattern changes and/or painful micturition.

Hip joint motion, flexion, extension, abduction, adduction, internal and external rotations are tested. Restrictions in any movement indicate pathology at the joint, e.g. arthritis or muscle contractures. Superficial and deep muscle palpation is conducted and painful points are located. Nerve tests are also conducted for each muscle group. Special tests such as *Trendelenburg test*, *Thomas test* and *Faber's test* are done to confirm specific pathologies. Laboratory tests like ESR, FBP, CRP and others are checked, especially in patients with symptoms other than pain, e.g. night sweating or fever. X-ray imaging in two planes, the antero-posterior (AP) and lateral views, are done to rule out fractures and other radio-visible conditions. MRI is quite informative for soft tissue and vascular conditions revealing avascular necrosis of the femur head in its early stage. Labral tears, ligament and tendon tears are also diagnosed by MRI. Its downside is that it is an expensive medical test for both the patient and the service provider. Diagnostic ultrasound is a valuable and affordable means to diagnose tendinopathies.

Treatment of hip tendonitis is referenced back to chapter 2 treatment options of tendinopathies. Healing takes time- several months to even a year. Many patients are frustrated by the delay in returning to play.

3) Groin tendonitis

Groin tendonitis, a.k.a. adductor tendonitis or *groin pull/groin strain*, is repeated stress injuries of the muscles located in the inside of the thigh- the adductor muscles. Strenuous workouts can put a huge strain on adductor muscles. With fatigue and inadequate rest, the muscles and their tendons become even more irritated. Strenuous activity without warming up causes adductor tendons to have micro-trauma, as they do not get a chance to adapt to increasing levels of exercise. Direct contact, e.g. a hard tackle in a rugby game or hitting a soccer goal post or another participant's leg, may result in sudden groin pull. Groin strain is recognized by a sudden sharp pain in the groin, which requires one to stop activity. Hip joint movement worsens this pain. Often, in 24 hours, swelling and tenderness become obvious with a warm feel to the touch and/or skin discolorations. Any activity, including walking, causes severe pain.

Routine blood works and imaging tests are done. Pain relief should be started immediately and as always RICE method, analgesics, massage and other intermediate pain relieving methods are used. Stretches and exercises are conducted during rehabilitation; see under physiotherapy for stretch examples.

4) Hamstring tendonitis

The hamstring muscle is a complex of 3 separate muscles that share the same origin point at the distal area of the pelvis, but are inserted on 3 different locations at the back of the knee. The *semimembranous*, *semitendinous* and *biceps femoris* muscles are the complex makeup. The hamstring muscle is responsible for propelling the body forward with each stride, bending the knee and straightening the hip, and is mostly active in jumping and kicking. Like a car engine, the more miles it covers on the speedometer, the greater its chance of a breakdown. Hamstring tendonitis can affect one or both thighs with pain located at the medial or lateral back of the knee, and at times radiating to the calf muscles and/or thigh muscles. A high hamstring tendinopathy is also possible where pain occurs at the single origin site of the hamstring muscle complex. The tendon gets inflamed and degenerates. Pain is the major complaint of sufferers, which worsens at night. Reduced activity is not uncommon and any attempt to do hard work, exercise or training intensifies pain. Hamstring tendonitis affects athletes who spend over 90 minutes on intense training and/or field running during soccer practice. Factors contributing to hamstring tendonitis are:

- hamstring muscle tightness

- poor biomechanics and posture

- inadequate warm up

- fatigue

- wrong footwear

- incorrect training techniques

- muscle weakness or imbalance

- flat feet

The best treatment option for hamstring tendonitis is non-surgical treatment, though it may take months to recover - see chapter 2 for treatment options.

5) Quadriceps tendonitis

Quadriceps tendonitis is characterized by injury and inflammation to the quadriceps tendon. The quadriceps muscle is located on the anterior thigh compartment and is made up of 4 segments, which combine to form one huge tendon, v*astus lateralis, vastus meadialis, vastus intermedius* and *rectus femoris*. The quadriceps muscle originates from the pelvis and femur, attaches to the kneecap (patella) as the quadriceps tendon, and is part of the knee extensor mechanism that extends via the patella tendon to finally attach to the shin bone at the tibial tuberosity. Quadriceps tendonitis may occur in any age group, but is most common in older active individuals. In the UK, incidence is at 1.37/100 000 per year with mean ages of 50.5 in males and 51.7 in females. At the knee, tendonitis can be of any region of the extensor mechanism, where 65% affects the patella tendon, 25% the quadriceps tendon, and 10% the tendon attachment at the tibial tuberosity. Causes of quadriceps tendonitis include repetitive squatting, kicking, jumping, hopping and running; also common in sports that require acceleration and deceleration such as basketball and netball, with sports of inclined surfaces, e.g. uphill running and/or downhill included. Quadriceps tendon may also rupture partially and/or totally when a patient rapidly contracts the quadriceps muscle in a flexed knee position. This extends great force over the tendon, which may exceed the tendon's tensile strength, resulting in a tear. Anatomy of the tendon has a weak watershed zone about 1-2 centimeters superior to the patella and it is this region that is susceptible to rupture. Research that has been conducted in patients who have had a rupture, revealed that this area had hypoxic degeneration and had decreased collagen fiber thickness. Ruptures are frequent in over-40s with a peak age between the 6th and 7th decade, men being 4-8 times more affected than women, and in particular black men with over 10 times a greater risk in comparison to counterparts of other races. History is associated with sudden supra-patella pain associated with falling, followed by inability to use the knee extensor mechanism. Acute quadriceps tendonitis may occur upon landing from a height.

As with any tendonitis, pain located above the kneecap and the bottom thigh area in front are the main complaints, increasing upon knee extension against resistance. Joint stiffness may also be associated, with swelling and a feeling of the knee giving way during exercises. Stretching and/or squeezing the tendon elicit more pain. Diagnosis is by clinical and physical examination, though occasionally ultrasound, X-ray and MRI are required in severe conditions. A torn tendon may have a gap just above the patella, with failure in the extensor mechanism of the knee.

With appropriate physiotherapy and exercises, plus pain and inflammation relief, quadriceps tendonitis can settle. Major key components require abstaining from activities that elicit pain such as jumping and squatting. Braces and knee supports can be worn for temporary pain relief. The earlier the treatment, the earlier the patient can get back to activity. A no pain, no gain attitude can further damage the tendon, leading to a chronic form and/or an actual tendon tear. RICE method can be initiated at home, with over-the-counter NSAIDs simultaneously being taken. When this pain management does not suffice, injection of steroids or autologous blood can be done. Once the pain is relieved, physio stretches and exercises can be initiated - *see physio chapters*. Physio includes soft tissue massage, electrotherapy, joint mobilization, patella tapping, footwear advice, stretches and activity modification. With appropriate treatment and management, minor quadriceps tendonitis recovers in a few weeks, and several months for the chronic cases. Early surgery is recommended for tears. Delay is associated with tendon retraction, hence shortening and atrophy, which result in poor functional outcomes. 6 weeks immobilization is required post-surgery and activity may not return to the before-injury state. In 25-67% of cases long-term muscle weakness has been reported.

Tips

Take fresh sage leaves and crush them with a mortar and pestle. To a vessel, add the crushed leaves and apple cider vinegar. Boil the mixture after which you wait for it to cool to tolerable heat. Dip a cloth in the warm vinegar + sage leaves, wring it out, and apply at the top part of the knee over the quadriceps tendon. Place the cloth until it cools then repeat for three more times. If this proves to be hard work for you, you can substitute by drinking sage leaves herbal tea 2-3 times a day.

6) Patella tendonitis

The patella tendon connects the kneecap to the shin, attachment of which is at the tibial tuberosity. Together with the quadriceps tendon and quadriceps muscle, they straighten the knee during walking and running. The patella tendon, like any tendon, is a thick fibrous rope that connects muscle to bone, inflammation of which causes patella tendonitis. Patella tendonitis is commonly known as the *jumper's knee,* as it is common in athletes who do repetitive jumping, e.g. volleyball and basketball players. Patella tendinopathy, being the correct term for this condition, is a chronic state, which develops gradually and is characterized by micro-trauma and abnormal tendon thickening. Tendon tears can occur and require surgical intervention.

Symptoms are direct pain over the patella tendon, which is accompanied by swelling and tenderness. Knee movement can produce a crepitating sound directly above the patella tendon. Pain is associated with activity, though post-activity pain at rest is not uncommon. X-rays are performed to rule out any bone involvement and ultrasound to exclude patella bursitis. MRI as always is expensive, but is a very informative imaging test.

Treatment involves all possible tendon treatment options; refer to chapter 1, though surgery is indicated in patients with chronic pain and rupture.

7) The knee and below it

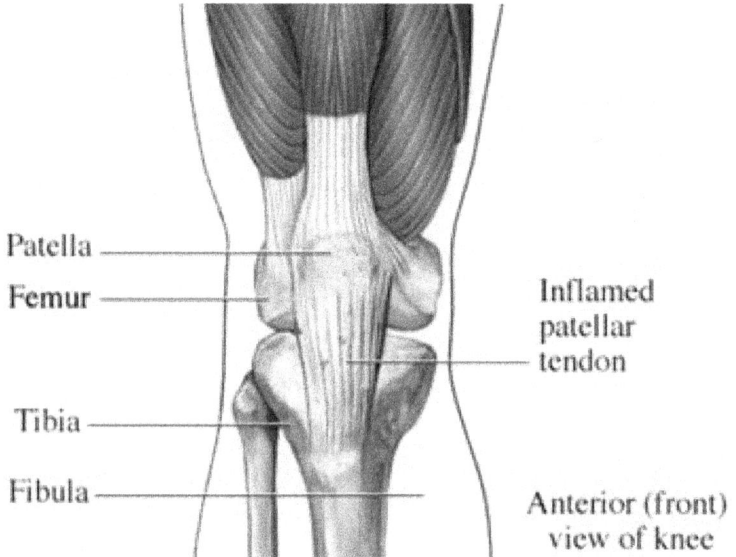

Anterior (front) view of knee

Patella
Femur
Tibia
Fibula
Inflamed patellar tendon

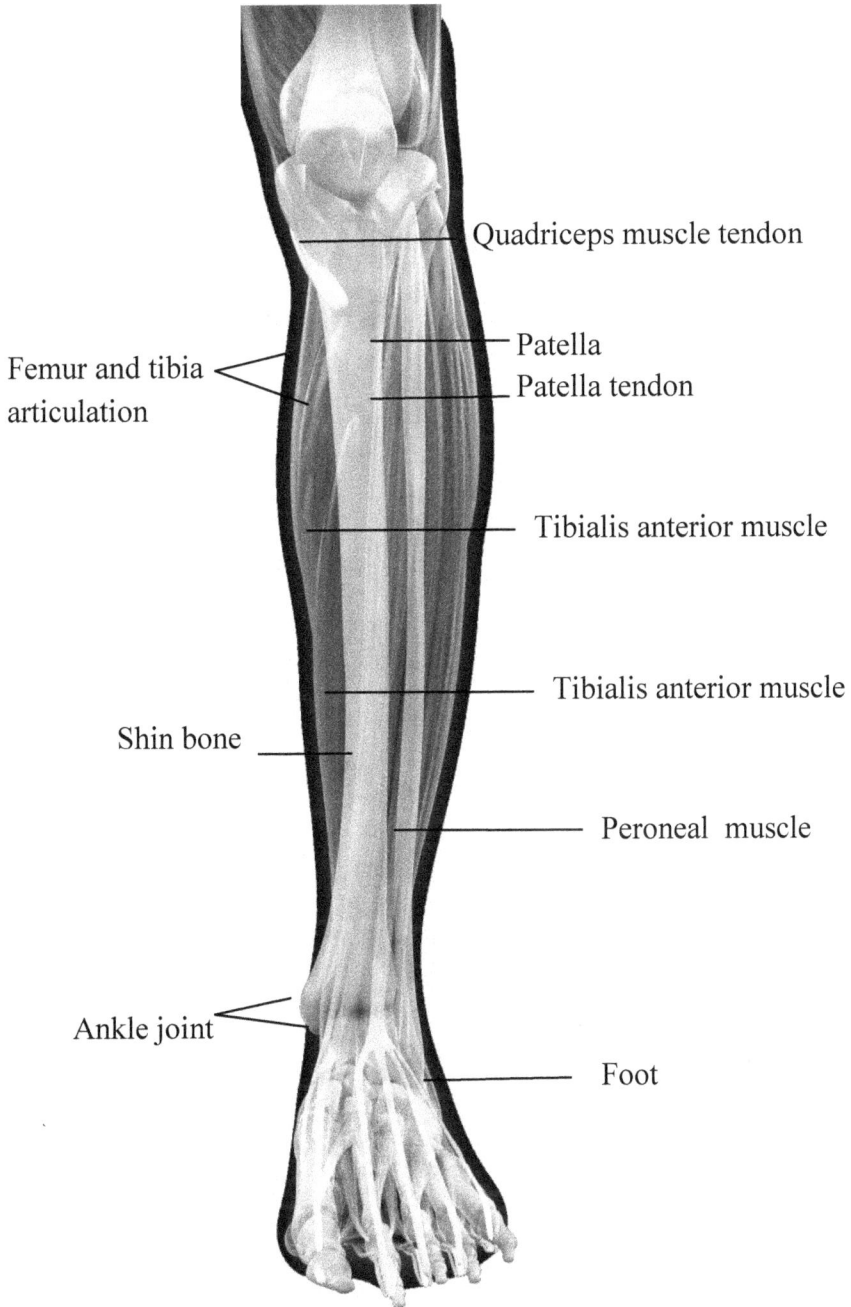

Quadriceps muscle tendon

Patella

Patella tendon

Femur and tibia
articulation

Tibialis anterior muscle

Tibialis anterior muscle

Shin bone

Peroneal muscle

Ankle joint

Foot

The knee is one of the biggest and most complex joints of the human body. It is an articulation of the femur and the shin bone (tibia). The fibula is close to the knee joint for support, but it does not articulate in the joint. The patella is the largest *sesamoid bone* of the body and is among the knee joint components as it sits on the femur to form the patella-femoral joint. The knee articulation is stabilized by ligaments and these are as follows:

ACL (anterior cruciate ligament) - it prevents the femur from sliding back on the tibia or the tibia sliding in front of the femur.

PCL (posterior cruciate ligament) - prevents back rolling of the tibia on the femur and forward femur riding over the tibia.

MCL (medial collateral ligament) - prevents sideways instability at the knee joint towards its inner surface.

LCL (lateral collateral ligament) - prevents sideways instability of the knee joint towards its outward surface.

Within the knee joint, which is a hinge joint, is a C-shaped rubbery shock absorber called the *meniscus*. This meniscus has 2 segments, the medial and lateral menisci. They absorb stress excited between the femur and the tibia. In the front of the knee are the quadriceps and patella tendons, which add stability to the joint. Between the patella tendon and the shin bone is a bursa that acts as a lubricant during movement. From behind the knee is a depression, the *popliteal fossa,* where nerves and blood vessels pass in close proximity to the bones. Posterior thigh muscles, the hamstrings, attach on the medial and lateral sides of the joint, also muscles on the back of the leg, e.g. gastrocnemius.

Besides hamstring tendonitis at the back, quadriceps and patella tendonitis in the front, knee pain has many differentials. Knee arthritis, which is caused by age, and cartilage damage is common. This arthritis can be of any kind, e.g. osteoarthritis, rheumatoid arthritis, gout arthritis, pseudo-gout and/or septic arthritis.

During inflammation the joint capsule may produce fluid above the normal quantity- resulting in a *joint effusion*. *Patella bursitis* is also common in inflammatory states and together with effusion is accompanied by swelling and visible fluid fluctuations. Meniscus tears may occur with trauma and patients complain of pain and joint catching associated with a popping sound as it is released. Any of the joint ligaments may rupture, leading to occurrence of joint instability, which the ligament protects against - e.g. ACL tear results in the femur sliding over the tibia. The patella position may be displaced in subluxation and/or dislocation, causing pain and disruption of gait. At the back a *Baker's cyst*, collection of joint fluid in a pocket, may cause pain.

Knee examination is clinical, physical and imaging. Manipulative tests, such as anterior and posterior drawers test, or varus and valgus stress tests may be conducted by a physician. X-rays, MRI and CT-scans are done with arthroscopy indicated in cases where imaging tests do not reveal any pathology. Joint fluid aspiration for therapeutic or diagnostic tests is often performed with consequent culturing and antibiotic spectrum deduction.

Below the knee is the leg, which is formed by 2 bones, the tibia and fibula, positioned parallel to each other running between the knee and ankle joints. Between these 2 bones is a fibrous tissue connecting them called a *syndesmosis*. The leg, like the forearm, consists of muscle compartments formed by fascial septa. 3 compartments of the leg are known. The anterior compartment has the muscles that pull the foot upwards (*dorsiflexion*) when they contract. These are *tibialis anterior muscle, extensor digitorum longus, extensor hallucis longus* and *peroneus tertias muscles*. The lateral compartment has the fibular muscles, named due to the close proximity of these muscles to the fibula bone. Fibular muscles are also called peroneal muscles because the peroneal nerve runs in this compartment. Within the lateral compartment are identified *peroneus longus and brevis muscles.*

When these muscles contract, they cause the foot to evert, like standing on the medial boarder of the foot. The posterior leg compartment is divided into superficial and deep, where the top lying muscles are the calf muscle balk, *gastrocnemius* and *soleus muscles*. The deep posterior compartment includes the *posterior tibialis muscle*, the *flexor digitorum* and *hallucis muscles*. These cause plantar flexion when they contract, as in tiptoe foot position. In each compartment run nerves and blood vessels responsible for supplying these muscles. Tendonitis can occur in any one tendon of these muscles with repetitive overuse. The most common kinds are described below.

8) Peroneal tendonitis

The lateral leg compartment contains the peroneal muscle group. The peroneal brevis muscle - the term brevis meaning short - is a short muscle which begins at the lower leg and runs around the back of the fibula where its tendon, together with the peroneal longus muscle tendon, pass in a groove bound by a retinaculum. The peroneal brevis tendon inserts at the fifth metatarsal. The long peroneal muscle has a longer course in comparison to the brevis - its tendon courses the fibula to insert on the first metatarsal. Overuse of these foot everters lead to strain and inflammation of their tendons at the back of the foot where pain and tenderness occurs in *peroneal tendonitis*. Peroneal tendonitis is caused by poor shoe quality and sporting activities that require use of the ankle, e.g. cross country running and marathons. This can increase with activity and is often not related to trauma. Peroneal tendonitis diagnosis is made by patient history where overuse, increased training and some sports with ankle function requirements are often reported. On physical examination, pain is located below the fibula end. Pain lying directly over the fibula may point to fracture of this bone, what is called the lateral malleolus. The lateral malleolus is the bony bump felt at the outside of the ankle. Peroneal tendons pass right behind this landmark. Moving the foot outwards may show lateral leg compartment muscle weakness and pain. Inward positioning of the heel often predisposes certain individuals to peroneal tendonitis - this should be checked during physical examination.

X-rays are done, though they are almost always normal. Ultrasound and MRI are effective in showing tendon tears. Most cases of peroneal tendonitis heal without surgery. Ankle braces and supports are worn to relieve pain. Crutches may be required to exempt the foot from weight bearing. Pain relieving treatment is initiated and physical therapy is of great importance. Stretches and exercises are done - see physiotherapy chapter for examples. If conservative treatment is not effective, surgery is indicated. Surgical procedures that are often carried out include deepening the peroneal tendon groove on the fibula. This increases space in which the tendons can move. If severe tendon injury exists, the affected tendon is resected and the 2 tendons joined, the peroneal longus and brevis tendons. Recovery is usually in full, though over a considerable amount of time. Outcomes are also good.

9) Tibialis posterior tendonitis

The tibialis posterior muscle is a constituent of the deep posterior compartment of the leg. Overuse of the muscle can result in posterior tibialis tendonitis. Posterior tibial tendon inflammation causes pain located at the inside of the ankle behind the bony bump- the lateral malleoulus. Tibialis posterior muscle originates from the top back of the tibia and fibula and runs along the inside of the lower leg and ankle where its tendon attaches to various bones of the foot. The posterior tibial muscle is responsible for inverting the foot, as in positioning the foot on its outer edge. This muscle tendon helps to maintain the arch of the foot and is active during walking and running. Posterior tibial tendonitis occurs in excessive running or walking, especially on steep bumpy surfaces. Patients with flat feet are predisposed to this condition. Poor shoe choices are also a contributing factor to its development. Athletes involved in hockey, athletics and speed skating are often affected by this condition. Pain behind the medial malleolus, experienced during walking or running, is typical. At times, swelling occurs over the tendon. Joint stiffness may also be associated. Pain is of gradual onset worsening over time. Diagnosis is by history, physical examination and imaging. See chapter 1 for tendon treatment options, with addition of shoe inserts and arch supports, walking boots and casts. In severe cases, the posterior tibialis tendon is replaced by its neighbouring tendon, the flexor digitorum longus tendon, in reconstructive surgery. If the foot arch is rigid, a fusion procedure is preferred. Though repair takes months or even a year, it is often complete.

Tips

While your tibialis posterior tendonitis heals, exercises that avoid lower leg strengthening can be performed, like stationery cycling, swimming, and current weight training.

10) Ankle tendonitis

The ankle is a hinged joint, capable of movement in two planes: dorsiflexion, as in moving the foot up towards the body, and plantar flexion, downward foot movement away from the body. This joint is formed by the articulation of 3 bones, the shin bone (tibia), fibula and foot bone (talus). The shin bone is located on the inside of the ankle and the fibula on the outside. These two bones form the ankle malleoli. The ankle is a body weight bearer during walking and running and is stabilized by ligaments that connect this bone to that bone. Like the knee, medial and lateral collateral ligaments are known among others. The ligaments are continuous with the joint capsule, which produces synovial fluid for lubrication. The Achilles tendon, being the largest, is located behind the lower leg and attaches to the calcaneus (heel bone), posterior tibialis tendon behind the medial malleolus and peroneal tendons at the back of the lateral malleolus. Pain at the ankle can arise due to many reasons. Sprains are by far the most common, resulting from ankle ligament injury. Fractures at the ankle are also common with tendonitis as another source of pain. Arthritis, nerve compression (*tarsal tunnel syndrome*), infections and synovitis are named among other reasons. Ankle tendonitis involves peroneal tendonitis, posterior tibialis tendonitis and Achilles tendonitis. *Refer to their individual descriptions for more information.*

11) Achilles tendonitis

Achilles tendon, or sometimes called Achilles heel, has been well-known since ancient times in Greek mythology where Achilles was the bravest and strongest warrior of the Trojan War. The myth says that when Achilles was a baby, his mother Thetis, in an attempt to make him immortal, dipped him into the principal underwater river, the *Styx.* Upon dipping him, she was holding him by the heel such that this area missed being dipped into the Styx, hence missing the magical immortal power and rendering it vulnerable. Achilles became the bravest warrior, as his mother had wanted. During his time it is said that he took 12 nearby cities. One day, quarrelling with the commander of the Greek forces, Agamemnon, who had invaded Troy, Achilles declined to further participate in war.

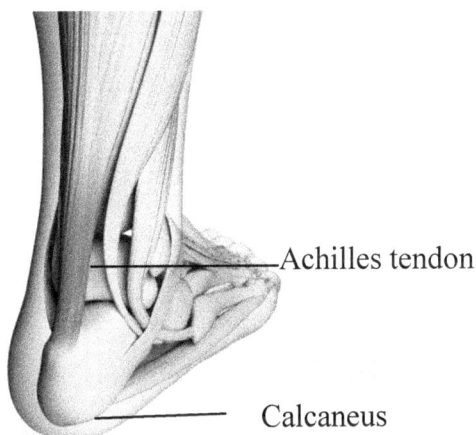

Achilles tendon

Calcaneus

After Achilles was forced to return to battle after the death of Patrochus, his cousin, who was killed by a Trojan warrior, Hector. Hector did not live long after this; he suffered the wrath of Achilles. It is said that Achilles was later killed by Paris, the prince of the Trojans, using an arrow guided by Apollo into his vulnerable heel. Since then, Achilles tendon is considered a vulnerable point in any individual, which anyone hit by a shopping cart would know. A novel of Achilles is available, written by Elizabeth Cook in 2002.

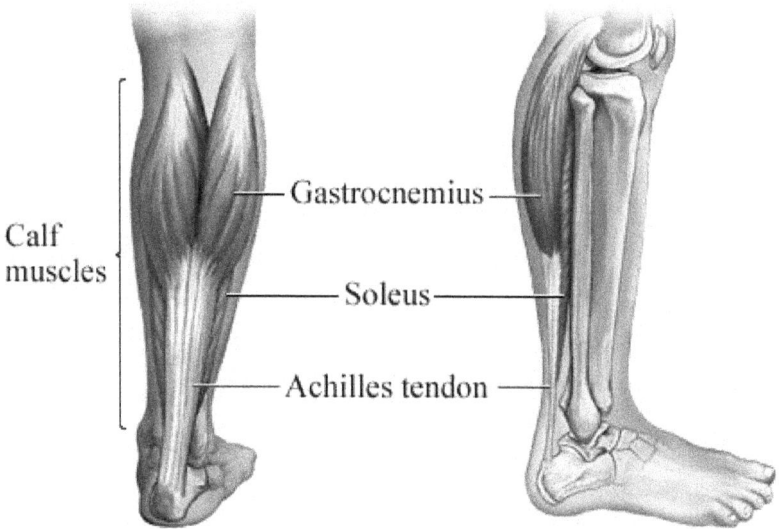

Calf muscles

Gastrocnemius

Soleus

Achilles tendon

The name "Achilles tendon" has been used since 1885 and means a fibrous band formed by the cuff muscles of the leg (*gastrocnemius, soleus* and *plantaris* muscles), attaching them to the heel bone, the *calcaneus*. These muscles, when they contract, cause the foot to point downwards like in tiptoeing, what is called *plantar flexion*. Plantar flexion is necessary for walking and is part of the swing phase of any stride. If the Achilles tendon is completely torn, one will lose the ability to plantar flex, hence to walk, run and tiptoe. These are functions that literally define your movement from one point to another, without which mobility is grossly impaired.

Like in any tendonitis, Achilles tendonitis involves the injury of the tendon due to repetitive stress, including inflammation and tendinosis. Achilles tendonitis often occurs in athletes such as runners, jumpers and even professionals who are always on their feet. Shoe choices too can contribute to its development. Achilles tendonitis is very common, occurring at seven times more in men than women, partly because men tend to be more involved in physical activities which require the tendon's function. Other reasons contributing to its occurrence include intensifying a training regimen, training on a hard or slopping surface, an underdeveloped or weak calf muscle and a high foot arch. *Psoriatic arthritis* and *ankylosing spondylitis* have been shown to occur with Achilles tendonitis. Two types of Achilles tendinopathy exist depending on what tendon area is affected. Insertional and non-insertional tendonitis are known. Insertion, as we understand, is the point at which a tendon attaches- in this case of Achilles the calcaneus. *Insertional tendonitis* involves pain at the tendon attachment point and can occur in any individual even those who are non-active. A great number of insertional tendonitis patients also have calcifications and bony spurs at this site. *Non-insertional tendonitis* occurs in those who are active and young, affecting the middle tendon region.

Achilles tendinopathy symptoms are pain and stiffness of a gradual development, which is generally worse in the morning. Pain is also worse after exercise though other sufferers feel it during activity. Severe, sudden pain may point out to an Achilles tendon rupture and requires an urgent doctor's consultation. Early tendon anastomosing or suturing is recommended in surgical principles if void of contraindications. *Thompson test* can be done to confirm a ruptured tendon. With a patient lying by the abdomen and the knee in a half bent position, squeezing the cuff muscles will result in the foot moving upwards (plantar flexion), this effect is absent in tendon rupture. Also, a patient may be asked to straighten their ankle which is not possible in a tendon rupture. A doctor might ask a patient to stand on tiptoes, which will elicit severe pain in the case of Achilles tendinopathy, failure of which diagnoses a tendon rupture. Achilles tendon swells up to form a bump or may creak when touched or moved. A doctor's physical examination may reveal enlargement of the Achilles tendon, a point of maximum tenderness and ankle limited range of motion, especially the ability to plantar flex. X-rays and other tests may be required to confirm diagnosis, ultrasound and MRI are quite informative tendon tests. Treatment of Achilles, like any other tendon is divided into non-surgical and surgical.

Non-surgical treatment

Prevention is better than cure they say. Achilles tendonitis can be prevented by alternating exercises, e.g. one day you jog, another you swim, this allows on and off tension on the tendon which gives it time to rest. Limiting exercises like hill running or a very steep treadmill reduces strain on the tendon. Arch supports in shoes are also helpful; they put off weight from the tendon. Stretching before an exercise is recommended with gradual increase of workout intensity plan. Wearing proper shock absorbing shoes reduces the chance of a tendonitis occurring.

In the case that Achilles tendonitis has already occurred, primary pain relief and anti-inflammatory medications are required. This is achieved by;

Rest - decreasing activities that elicit pain and cross training is easy on the tendon.

Ice - using ice to relieve swelling is helpful and can be done as often as required, taking care not to apply ice directly to skin.

Non-steroidal anti-inflammatory drugs - e.g. ibuprofen reduce swelling and pain. Long-term use however should be reviewed by a physician.

Exercises- stretch and strengthening exercises improve tendon function and reduce stress.

Orthotics and shoe support - e.g. braces and arch support put weight off the tendon.

Physiotherapy and intermediary pain relief managements, such as cortisone injections and shockwave therapy are some other means available.

Surgical intervention

6 months of no relief from non-surgical management should have a consideration for surgery and/or tendon rupture. Many surgical interventions are available for Achilles tendonitis treatment. They are dependent on location of the tendonitis and extent of the injury.

If a tendon has less than 50% injury, debridement and repair can be done. This involves excision of all unhealthy tendon tissues; the remaining healthy bit is repaired by sutures. This includes excision of bony spurs in insertional tendonitis. After repair, a patient is placed in a post-surgery boot for 2weeks. In cases where tendon damage is more than 50%, tendon transfer after debridement is performed. Debridement is done to remove the damaged tendon part; the remaining has weak strength and is at great risk of rupturing. Another tendon, usually that of the great toe is transferred and attached to the heel for added strength. Some patients cannot plantar flex due to a tight Achilles tendon. An elongation operation can be done. Elongation is possible as an open surgery and/or as a minimal invasive scope procedure.

In most cases, patients have good results after surgery. Physiotherapy is implemented after 4-6weeks post-surgery. Rarely do complications occur, pain has been reported in about 30% of cases and infection, when it occurs, is very difficult to eradicate.

Tips

Try the Arctic ease cryotherapy wrap on your tendonitis. It can be used on the ankle, elbow, wrist, shoulder, and even on a jumper's knee, available from Amazon.com, Walgreens.com, and drugstore.com. Sitting while you ice your ankle can be a bit boring; the Arctic ease wrap allows walking and stretching while you ice. It sticks in place without moving and remains cold for hours. Icing an Achilles tendonitis is controversial, as some reports focus on heat treatment and not ice. This can also be explained by sufferers who improve on heat treatment in comparison to cold and vice versa. If one gives you no relief, try the other.

12) Foot tendonitis

The foot is a separate organ at the end of the leg, like the hand is for the forearm. It is made up of segments, which are divided into hind, mid and fore foot. The hind foot is composed of the heel bone (calcaneus) and the ankle bone (talus), articulating with each other at the subtalar joint. The mid foot is made up of 5 bones that are irregular in shape, the *cuboid, navicular* and 3 *cuneiform bones.* These bones form the arch of the foot and act as shock absorbers. The fore foot is composed of 5 long bones *(metatarsals)*, which connect to 5 toes. Like the fingers of the hand, the big toe has two segments whereas the other 4 toes have 3 segments each. These bones are covered by ligaments and muscles and act as anchor sites for tendons of the leg muscles. Intrinsic and extrinsic muscles of the foot are named. The top foot surface is called the *dorsum foot* and the bottom is referred to as the plantar. Pain in the foot can occur if one or more of its components are injured. Arthritis is the leading cause in above 40s with rheumatoid arthritis, gout and osteoarthritis being the common types. *Plantar fasciitis* is frequent- inflammation of the fascia ligament at the bottom of the foot. Pain is felt in the heel and the arch of the foot. Diabetic foot is a complication of diabetes, which requires prevention, as many have been amputated because of it. Corns, mallet toes, claw toes, bunions, swollen feet and fractures are among other foot pain causes. Physical examination and imaging tests are used to differentiate the diagnosis.

Foot tendonitis occurs due to strain of the foot in activities such as running and walking. It is the inflammation, degeneration and/or tear of the tendons of the foot. Tendons involved in foot tendonitis are the peroneal tendon, posterior tibialis tendon, anterior tibialis tendon and Achilles tendon *(refer to their individual tendonitis descriptions).* Symptoms of foot tendonitis include pain and a burning sensation. Treatment is as any other tendonitis type, this also is referenced to individual tendon descriptions.

Tips

Foot tendonitis can be relieved by soaking. Many soakings have been deemed effective, and we have a list of tips for you to try.

1) A contrast bath can be refreshing for hurting feet due to tendonitis. A contrast bath involves filling a tab with cold water and soaking your feet for 10-15 minutes. Replace the cold water with warm water and soak your feet again for 10 minutes. Lastly, a cold water soak is done for yet another 10 more minutes. This can be repeated as many times as you can.

A different twist to contrast soaking is warm and cold vinegar wrapping. In this technique, warm a mixture of half part water and vinegar, and then, pour it in a basin. In another basin, put half part cold water and vinegar. Soak a cloth in the cold vinegar-water mixture and wring it out. Wrap your foot with the cloth for 5 minutes. Then, dip the same cloth in the warm vinegar-water mixture. Wring it out and wrap your foot again for 5 minutes. Repeat the procedure with the cold mix one more time.

2) Soak your feet in carbonated water for 10-15 minutes instead of normal water.

3) Soak your feet in Epsom salt. Use 2-3 tablespoons of Epsom in a basin of warm water. Then, dip your feet for 10 minutes. Epsom salt contains magnesium sulphate, which replenishes foot cells upon soaking. Apply moisturizer after an Epsom salt soak; it has a tendency to dry feet.

For runners, take note of a persistent localized pain. It should be differentiated from a stress fracture; an x-ray will do the trick. Deep tissue massage, as well as energy healing modalities, like Jin Shin Jyutsu, acupressure, and Shiatsu, can be effective if the correct professional performs them. If massage is done at home, try using warm olive oil.

Chapter 5) Physiotherapy

1) What is physiotherapy?

Physiotherapy, also known as physical therapy, is a branch of medicine involving diagnosis and treatment of medical conditions using physical means. Physiotherapists, or physical therapists, practice this conventional medicine. Physiotherapy offers a wide range of treatment options from massage to electric shock therapy among many other modalities. It is dedicated to maximizing patient's mobility and function. In general, it promotes physical activity, prevents disability, manages acute and chronic conditions, improves patient self-dependence, rehabilitates injuries through therapeutic programs and educates and advises patients. All this physical therapy will no doubt improve health, lifestyle and the quality of life.

Physiotherapy does not concentrate only on tendonitis rehabilitation. Its practice areas include:

Chronic care – in patients who suffer from stroke, heart disease or arthritis, physiotherapy maintains joint function, flexibility and helps in managing pain.

Sports physiotherapy – sprains, strains, ligament tears, tendonitis and muscle pathologies benefit from this branch of medicine without which these structures deteriorate if they are not physically challenged.

Incontinence treatment – physiotherapy includes bladder and bowel control exercises. This is very important in spinal cord injury patients or in patients who have had prostate surgery.

Neurologic conditions – such as cerebral palsy, Parkinson's disease and multiple sclerosis respond to specialized physiotherapy programs, since these patients need to relearn motor function.

In orthopaedics, physiotherapists are part and parcel of this specialty, where almost all patients require physiotherapy, e.g. arthritic patients, those with back pain, joint injuries and muscle problems. Physiotherapists work in hospitals, outpatient clinics, sports clubs and can even visit patients in the comfort of their own home. These professionals are required to develop a long-term relationship with a patient, since the treatment plans they offer require several sessions, and the conditions that they deal with are chronic and take a long time to respond to treatment. Even if they do respond, physio in most cases is still required to maintain the achievement and to prevent relapses.

Physiotherapists can be accessed through the NHS or via private practice. Although other routes exist, like charities and voluntary sectors. To see a physiotherapist you can ask your doctor or the local NHS hospital for directions, although self-referral systems are in place.

2) Tendonitis - Where to get help

Information in this book is not a substitute to doctors' advice. Your physician is the first person to turn to in any medical complaint. Doctors will check your history, clinical signs and symptoms, and will examine you physically using special stress tests to confirm certain phenomena. Your doctor will also order laboratory and imaging tests to confirm the diagnosis and/or differentiate conditions. This is important, as any immediate disease states are diagnosed early. Consequently, treatment is initiated early before any complications develop. Making an appointment directly with a specialist is another way to get help. For tendonitis, sports medicine specialists, orthopaedicians, physical therapists and specialists of the region of your interest, e.g. hand specialists for hand tendonitis, may be consulted.

The Internet is a great tool to research anything. One can research the type of tendonitis that they are interested to learn more about. Understanding your condition is helpful, as you discover some helpful tips in the process. A vast array of websites are in place, an example being www.nhs.uk. On this website, one can search for tendonitis. Many information sites pop up, e.g. a list of over-the-counter medicines that can be used for tendonitis, a list of ongoing clinical trials for tendonitis and tendonitis as a medical condition with its regional differentials. Other sites with tendonitis information are www.orthopedics.about.com, www.webmd.com and www.orthoinfo.aaos.org, to mention but a few. Books that are centered on tendonitis are also excellent choices to gather information. Some books available on the market are "Treat your own Achilles tendinitis" and "Treat your own rotator cuff," both by Jim Johnson, available on Amazon. Also on Amazon is "Cure yourself of tendinitis, volume 1." www.barnesandnoble.com is another website where you can check many other books on sale.

One can also join discussion groups where tendonitis sufferers share their experiences, things they find effective and those that are a waste of time. This can prevent repeating the same mistakes, but then again the Internet as we know it, is full of diverse people, from genuine people who really want to share their opinions and experiences, to scammers who just want you to buy their products and/or medicines. It is difficult to differentiate these people, because all actually seem genuine. One is required to develop a sixth sense to prevent falling for the same tricks that many others have before. Discussion groups that you could check out are www.patient.co.uk/forums, www.banjohangout.org, forums.webmd.com, www.orthogate.org, for swimmers, forums.usms.org, and forums.military.com. On forums.military.com, you can also check some different fitness techniques and tips, workouts and nutrition.

Once the correct diagnosis of tendonitis has been made by your physician you are, however, not required to see the physiotherapists very frequently. You can learn how to do the physio routines correctly in the first sessions with your physiotherapist, after which you can continue the program from home. Other pain and inflammation-relieving treatments can be done from home as well, the likes of the RICE method, bracing and use of joint supports. NSAIDs can be bought over-the-counter from your local pharmacy.

Chapter 6) Stretches and exercises for different kinds of tendonitis

1) How to exercise with tendonitis

Tendonitis is not easy to deal with. It takes time, effort and willingness to try this and that since treatment plans are often in combination with switching and swapping between different available methods. No one method exists to cure tendonitis at a go. Exercise routines maintain function, rehabilitate injuries and strengthen. However, a wrong exercise technique can cause further damage. This is why it is always important to consult with your physician and/or physiotherapist before starting any physio routines and/or programs. Exercise also needs to be initiated at an optimal time, which also needs consultation with a physical therapist to be told when to start exercising. Tendonitis often affects the shoulder, knee, elbow, heel and wrist, among other locations. Once your doctor gives a green light to exercise, since your tendons have been injured and also have been non-functional for several days due to the initial rest protocol after injury, initial exercise necessitates that you begin slowly with stretches and not push yourself too hard. Your exercise should not include the motion that resulted in your tendonitis in the first place and should not be conducted through pain. Continuing through pain can further damage tendons. Remember, pain is the body's way of notifying you about tissue injury.

In the absence of pain, exercise can proceed, making sure that routines are varied and not to concentrate on a single stretch over and over - this can cause a new repetitive injury in a different location and/or a relapse. Warming up before exercise is recommended - this generates heat within muscles, tendons and the body in general. Cold conditions have been shown to increase the probability of tendon injury. Warming up also prepares the muscles and body for a step in speed, weight and function. An abrupt switch or change of gear often results in tears. After exercise, stretches are also recommended. In this case, they allow your body to rest with ease and at the same time, prepares tendons for your next exercise session. At times, initiating exercise routines can result in flare-ups. A flare-up is exacerbation of tendonitis, with symptoms of tendonitis appearing such as pain, swelling, warmth and tingling sensations in some regions. This, however, does not mean a new condition has started and/or your tendonitis has worsened. If it occurs, stop exercising and initiate the usual tendonitis treatment protocol. Ice packs to cool off the area, with immobilization in a splint, brace or support and NSAIDs can also be taken. When the flare-up subsides, you can try the routine again. The bottom line to tendonitis exercise programs is not to push yourself overboard, to allow your body to adapt and heal, and to follow your physician's advice before starting any activity and/or to return to normal workouts. With that said, check out some of our tendonitis exercises by tendonitis type.

2) Rotator cuff exercises

Rotator cuff stretches and range of motion routines restore flexibility. Strength-building routines will stabilize the shoulder.

a) The pendulum swing

1) Hold the back of a chair with the normal hand.

2) Bend your body forward a bit and let the affected arm hang straight down.

3) Move the hanging arm back and forth like a pendulum for 2 minutes.

4) Then, move the hanging arm in circles, starting with smaller circles increasing the circle size, in anticlockwise direction, then in clockwise direction.

5) Do this for 5 minutes, about 5 times a day.

Tips

As your shoulder improves, this stretch can be intensified by holding a 0.5-1 kg weight in the swinging hand, a dumbbell or a bottle filled with water.

b) Crossing over arm stretch

1) Place one arm straight across your chest as far as possible.

2) Use the other arm to hold the crossing arm in position for 30 seconds.

3) Relax for 30 seconds and repeat the process with the other arm.

4) Repeat this 5 times on each side for 5-8 times a day.

Tip

Do not pull the elbow on step 2.

c) Isometric rotator cuff stretch

1) Stand sideways against a wall.

2) Bend the elbow in contact with the wall to 90°.

3) Press this arm against the wall, contracting your muscles for 4 seconds (keep your shoulder still as you do this).

4) Relax for 4 seconds and repeat the process 4 times.

5) Turn around and place the anterior or inside part of your forearm against the wall.

6) Repeat steps 3 and 4.

7) To be done 4-5 times a day.

d) Shoulder blade shrug

1) Stand with your back and neck in a straight position.

2) Place your arms on your side slightly away from your body, with your palms facing forward.

3) Raise one shoulder towards the ear as far as possible.

4) Hold the shrug for 5 seconds.

5) Release and repeat 8-10 times on each side.

6) To be done 5 times a day.

e) Sleeping stretch

1) Lie on a flat surface with your side, the affected shoulder, under you.

2) Place the elbow in a bent position with the forearm in a standing position.

3) Use the normal hand to push the affected arm down until you feel a stretch at the back of the affected shoulder.

4) Hold this position for 30 seconds.

5) Rest for 30 seconds and repeat 4-5 times, about 6 times a day.

Tip

Do not bend at the wrist and/or press down at the wrist.

f) Dumbbell elbow flexion stretch

For this exercise, you will require small weight dumbbells, they can be bought from Amazon.com.

1) Stand straight with your feet together.

2) While holding a dumbbell in each hand, place your elbows close to your side.

3) On one side, slowly bring the dumbbell up towards your shoulder.

4) Hold the position for 4 seconds.

5) Slowly return the arm to starting position.

6) Do the same on the other arm.

7) Repeat 5 times on each side.

Tip

This exercise should not be done too quickly.

g) Dumbbell elbow extension stretch

1) Stand straight with an even distribution of weight over your feet.

2) Raise one arm straight up while holding a dumbbell.

3) Bend your elbow with the weight behind your head.

4) Slowly straighten your elbow to bring it overhead.

5) Repeat the process 5 times on each side.

h) Horizontal abduction stretch

1) Hold a small weight dumbbell with your affected arm.

2) Lie with your stomach on a table or bed, with the affected arm and dumbbell hanging over the edge.

3) Keeping your elbow straight, raise the dumbbell up to the level of your eyes.

4) Hold the position for 4 seconds.

5) Bring it down slowly to starting position.

6) Repeat 5 times.

i) Shoulder rotation stretch

1) Hold a small weight dumbbell with your affected arm.

2) Lie on your side with the normal shoulder tucked under your head.

3) Fixing your affected arm to your side, raise the dumbbell vertically in a slow motion.

4) Hold the position for 4 seconds.

5) Repeat 5 times.

Tip

For all the exercises that use a dumbbell, as your shoulder improves, the stretch can be intensified by increasing the size of the dumbbell weight - however, a gradual increase is recommended, e.g. from 0.5 kg to a 1 kg. Pushups over the wall and/or the floor can be added to strengthen the shoulder, when it is pain-free, flexible and has complete range of motion.

3) Bicipital tendonitis stretches

a) Biceps hammer stretch

1) Hold a hammer with your affected hand.

2) Bend your elbow to a 90° angle.

3) Keeping your elbow in a fixed position, move the hammer towards the left side.

4) Hold the position for 10 seconds.

5) Then, move the hammer towards the right, maintaining your grip on the hammer.

6) Hold this position also for 10 seconds.

7) Repeat left-right cycles 10 times.

8) Rest for 30 seconds and repeat the routine to make 3 sets.

b) Biceps towel stretch

1) Hold one end of a hand towel with your normal arm.

2) Throw it over your normal shoulder so that the towel hangs down your back.

3) Use your affected arm to reach up your back and grab the other end of the towel.

4) Pull the towel gently with your normal hand until you feel a stretch on the biceps of the affected side.

5) Hold this position for 10 seconds.

6) Rest for 4 seconds and repeat 10 times.

7) Repeat routine in 3 sets.

c) Bicep curls

1) Hold a light weight with your affected arm (a hammer, a can of food, a dumbbell or a bottle of water).

2) Stand with your back and head in a straight position.

3) With your elbow close to your body at a 90 ° angle, slowly raise your hand up to the level of your shoulder.

4) Hold the position for 10 seconds.

5) Slowly release the arm to the starting position.

6) Repeat the curl 5 times daily.

d) Biceps flexion stretch

1) Stand facing a wall.

2) Walk your affected arm up the wall, by placing your palm flat on its surface with each step.

3) As your hand gets higher above your head, you will feel a stretch on your arm and shoulder.

4) Hold the position for 10 seconds.

5) Move the arm down to the starting position and repeat the routine 10 times.

e) Broomstick internal rotation stretch

1) Hold a broomstick with both hands at either end, behind you, in a horizontal position.

2) While standing straight, slide the stick up until you feel a stretch at the front of the shoulders.

3) Hold for 10 seconds and return slowly to the starting position.

4) Repeat this exercise 5 times.

f) Broomstick flexion stretch

1) In a standing position, hold a broomstick with both hands at either end, in front of you, in a horizontal position.

2) With the normal arm, push the broomstick towards the affected side; this will raise the affected side up and over head.

3) A stretch is felt on the raised arm at the biceps and shoulder.

4) Hold the position for 10 seconds and slowly return to the resting position.

5) Repeat the routine 10 times.

4) Triceps tendonitis exercises

a) Triceps strengthening exercise

1) Hold a dumbell or a light weight with your affected arm.

2) Lie on your back with the affected arm and the weight pointing up towards the sky.

3) Bend your elbow completely, so that the weight is a bit shy to rest on your shoulder, and the is elbow pointing up.

4) Straighten your elbow to point the hand and weight up to the sky again.

5) Repeat 10 times.

6) Rest 30 seconds and repeat the routine to make 3 sets.

b) Triceps towel stretch

1) Hold one end of a hand towel with your affected arm.

2) Throw it over the shoulder on the affected side, so that the towel hangs down your back.

3) Use your normal arm to reach up your back and grab the other end of the towel.

4) Pull the towel down with your normal hand, until you feel a stretch on the triceps of the affected side.

5) Hold this position for 10 seconds.

6) Rest for 4 seconds and repeat 10 times.

7) Repeat the routine in 3 sets.

c) French stretch

1) Stand in a straight position.

2) Join your hands together, with fingers locked together.

3) Lift the locked hands up towards the sky.

4) Bring the clasped hands behind your head to stretch the triceps muscles (keep arms as close to the ears as possible).

5) Hold the position for 20 seconds.

6) Slowly return to the starting position.

7) Repeat 5-6 times.

d) French press

1) Hold a light weight with both of your hands as if you are holding a baseball bat.

2) Sit on a chair, with your back against the back rest.

3) Reach towards the ceiling with the weight using both hands.

4) Bend your elbow, slowly lowering the weight towards the back, until the weight touches your upper back.

5) Lift the weight back up again, while straightening your elbow.

6) Repeat these presses 10-20 times.

e) Triceps kick back

1) With your normal arm, hold the back of a chair for support.

2) Bend your body forward, halfway, letting the affected arm (which is holding a light weight) hang beside you.

3) Bend your elbow to a 90 ° angle, with your upper arm parallel to the floor.

4) Move your forearm backwards to stretch the triceps and hold for 4 seconds.

5) Release and repeat this back and forth motion 10-20 times.

5) Tennis elbow stretches

a) Wall tennis elbow stretch

1) Stretch both arms in front of you.

2) Place your hands, palms facing forward, to rest on the wall surface (fingers should be pointing up).

3) Lift the base of your palm, so that top half part of the palm is still attached to the wall.

4) Press down gently on the fingers, like a press up.

5) Hold position for 4 seconds.

6) Release and repeat press ups 10 times.

b) Tennis ball squeeze

1) Use the affected arm to hold a tennis ball.

2) Tightly squeeze the ball 20-25 times.

3) Rest for 30 seconds and repeat routine to make 3 sets.

Tip

This exercise can be done with increased or reduced intensity. Use a sponge, or something softer if your elbow is tender, or a hard piece of rubber for a more intense tennis elbow stretch.

c) Rubber band stretch

1) Place a rubber band over your fingers and thumb.

2) Stretch the rubber band by opening your fingers wide.

3) Repeat the stretch 20 times in 3 sets, 5 times a day.

Tip

The intensity of this exercise depends on the quality of the rubber band. The more stiff or tense the band is, the more intense the stretch will be; however, begin with a very soft band and pave your way up to a more stiff band.

Do not *start with a very tense rubber band, it may cause more damage to your elbow.*

d) Broomstick elbow stretch

1) Using the affected arm, grip a broomstick on its middle.

2) Place the broomstick in front of you, in a vertical position.

3) Move the broomstick forward, without changing your grip, so that it lies in a horizontal position.

4) Hold the position for 4 seconds, then bring it back up.

5) Repeat the process 10 times.

Tip

As your tennis elbow improves, shift your grip on the broomstick step by step, towards the bottom end. The more your grip is distal on the broomstick, the more weight exerted on your elbow by the stretch.

e) Resistance band therapy

A resistance band can be found on Amazon.com. It is a thick elastic rope with handles on both ends.

1) Using the affected hand, hold both handles of the resistance band.

2) Using the mid foot of the same side as the affected arm, step over the loop of the rope to prevent it from sliding during exercise.

3) Place the affected hand straight in front and parallel to the knee with the hand in a fist.

4) Place the normal hand above the fist of the affected side.

5) Let the wrist of the affected side slowly drop towards the ground over 4 seconds.

6) Use the overlying normal hand to pull the affected hand back up to its starting position.

7) Let go of the normal hand and allow the affected hand to drop again, slowly, towards the ground. This marks a single rotation.

8) Repeat the process to make 15 rotations, in 3 sets, about 5 times a day.

Tip

Shortening the resistance band and using a stiffer rope intensifies this exercise.

6) Golfer's elbow exercises

a) Gofer's elbow stretch

1) Place your affected arm straight in front of you, with your palm facing forward like a policeman stopping a car.

2) Rotate your hand in a clockwise direction if it is the right side and counterclockwise for left, until your fingers are facing downwards.

3) With your normal hand, pull the down pointing fingers towards you in a moderate stretch.

4) Hold the position for 30 seconds.

5) Release the hold and repeat 5 times.

6) To be done 3-5 times a day.

b) Advanced elbow stretch

1) Place the affected arm over a table with the palm facing up and the wrist hanging over the table edge.

2) Using the normal hand, stretch the fingers down the edge of the table as far as you can.

3) Hold the position for 20 seconds and release.

4) Repeat the routine 10-20 times.

c) Massage

1) Palpate the inside of the affected elbow to locate the most tender spot.

2) Using the index and the middle finger of the normal side, apply firm pressure over this tender spot.

3) Rub in circular motion for 5 minutes.

4) Repeat this routine as often as required.

d) Flexion and extension

1) Place your normal hand in a fist on the palm of the affected side.

2) With the affected side, grip the normal fist tightly.

3) Move the normal side's wrist using your affected side back and forth, against resistance.

4) Repeat this process 20 times.

Tip

Also, for golfer's elbow, the rubber band stretch, tennis ball squeeze, and biceps hammer stretch can be done.

7) Forearm exercises for tendonitis

a) Reverse curls

1) Hold a light weight with the affected arm (e.g. a dumbbell).

2) Place your arm straight, next to your body, with the forearm facing backwards.

3) Bend your elbow to bring the weight towards your shoulder.

4) Concentrate on your forearm, moving the weight up to the shoulder and down to the starting position.

5) Repeat this reverse curl 10 times.

Tip

A reverse curl is like a bicep curl, though the arm position is facing backwards.

b) Fist clench

1) Using the affected arm, bend at the elbow to a 90° angle.

2) Clench your hand into a tight fist, feeling the forearm muscles tightening.

3) Move the fist towards you and down (moving only at the wrist), to feel the forearm muscles tighten even further.

4) Rotate the forearm, so that the wrist faces forward, and you bend at the wrist towards you. (Feel the muscles at the back of the forearm tighten).

5) Repeat this process 10 times on each side (i.e. the front and back muscle groups of the forearm).

8) Wrist physio stretches

a) Wrist roll

1) Using the affected hand, extend the wrist in front of you.

2) The palm should be facing down.

3) Slowly rotate your wrist in a clockwise direction for 30 seconds.

4) Switch the rotation to counterclockwise direction for another 30 seconds.

5) Repeat 4 times.

b) Wrist tendon lubricating glides

1) Using the affected arm, hold your hand out in front of you, palm facing down.

2) Use the normal hand to slowly pull each finger towards the palm.

3) Each finger should touch 2 areas: the middle of the palm and the bottom of the palm, starting with the pinky.

4) When you reach the thumb, cross it over to touch the base of the pinky.

5) Repeat this routine 3 times a day.

Tip

This exercise helps lubricate tendons at the wrist.

c) Grip devices

1) Grab a grip ball with the affected hand.

2) Squeeze it repeatedly 20-25 times.

Tip

This exercise is good to strengthen the wrist and to improve hand function. It requires you to use grip balls and grip levers, which can be bought from Amazon.com and body building websites.

d) Wrist radial and ulnar deviation

1) Using the affected side, stretch your hand, palm facing down, in front of you.

2) Bend your hand and wrist to one side, and hold the position for 4 seconds.

3) Then, bend the wrist and hand towards the other side, again holding for 4 seconds.

4) Repeat the routine 8-12 times.

e) Wrist flexion and extension

1) Using the affected arm, place the forearm facing down on a table with the wrist extended over the table edge.

2) With the forearm fixed, move your hand up, forming a fist as you do so, and hold the position for 4 seconds.

3) Then, lower your hand down the table edge, unclenching the fist, and let your fingers free, and again hold this position for 4 seconds.

4) Repeat 8-10 times.

9) Hand tendonitis exercises

a) Open hand stretch

1) Hold the affected hand, palm facing down, in front of you.

2) Keep your fingers together, though not tensed.

3) Spread your fingers out as far as possible and hold the position for 30 seconds.

4) Relax your hand and repeat the process 4 times.

b) Paper crumple stretch

1) Hold the affected hand, palm facing up in front of you.

2) Take a piece of paper, and slowly crumple it, with your ill hand, into a ball.

3) Clench your fist tightly to squeeze the paper in your hand.

4) Keep your fist clenched for 10 seconds.

5) Unclench your fist and rest for 10 seconds.

6) Clench your fist again for 10 seconds and release.

7) Repeat the routine, using a new piece of paper every time, 3-5 times.

10) Hip exercises

a) Half circles

1) Hold a table, a chair or a counter with the hand opposite to your affected side.

2) Stand on the normal leg, in a straight position with your pelvis still.

3) Let your affected leg hang in a straight position.

4) Rotate the leg in a clockwise direction 15 times.

5) Then rotate the leg in a counterclockwise direction 15 times.

6) Relax for 5 seconds and repeat another set.

b) Leg lifts

1) Lie straight on your normal side.

2) With a straight leg, lift your affected side up slowly as far as you can.

3) Bring it down to its starting position.

4) Repeat this leg lift 15 times, then switch to the other leg.

Tip

This exercise can be done with the knees bent.

c) Butterfly stretch

1) Sit on the floor, with your back straight.

2) Bend the knees and place the soles of your feet together.

3) Hold your feet with both of your hands and slowly push down on your knees with your elbows.

4) Hold position for 20-30 seconds.

5) Release and repeat 5 times.

d) Back kick

1) Hold a counter or a table with both hands for support.

2) Keep your body in a straight position.

3) Stretch your affected leg in a straight position, behind you, as far as you can.

4) Hold the position for 6 seconds

5) Release slowly and repeat.

e) Hip flexion

1) Stand straight with your normal side next to a chair or a table.

2) Hold the chair or table for support.

3) Bending at the knee, lift the affected leg up as far as you can.

4) Hold the position for 5 seconds.

5) Release and repeat 5 times.

11) Quadriceps exercises

a) Step up

1) Using a stool or elevated surface, approximately 6 inches above the ground, step up with your affected leg.

2) Step down, and then up again, 20-30 times.

3) Rest for 30 seconds and repeat to make another set.

b) Wall squat with a ball

1) Place a basketball or a soccer ball behind your back, and press it against the wall

2) Slide down at 45 degrees, and hold the position for 15 seconds.

3) Slide back up and repeat 10 times.

C) Jogging in water

1) In a swimming pool, jog on the same spot 20-30 times.

2) Rest for 30 seconds, and repeat another set of 20.

Tip

Jogging in water works your quadriceps tendon especially as rehabilitation post-surgery. The water relieves stress on the knee and allows quadriceps muscles to be stretched properly.

12) Patella tendonitis stretch routine

a) Double leg squat

1) Stand with your feet spread apart.

2) Place your hands on your hips, with your back straight.

3) Drop slowly into an almost sitting position.

4) Hold this position for 6 seconds, and come back up.

5) Repeat squat 10 times, 2 times a day.

b) Quads over falcrum

1) Lie flat on your back.

2) Use a folded towel, or a small blanket under the knee to raise the affected leg approximately 4-6 inches off the ground.

3) Relax your knee and let your leg drop over the rolled towel or blanket.

4) Tighten your quadriceps muscle, and raise the leg, with your foot at a 90° angle, to the shin bone.

5) Hold your leg up for 6 seconds.

6) Repeat exercise 10 times.

c) Static quadriceps contraction

1) Lie flat on your back, on the floor.

2) Apply a round pillow or a rolled towel under your affected leg at the knee.

3) Contract the quadriceps muscle, while pressing your knee on the pillow or towel, as hard as you can.

118

4) Hold the position for 6 seconds.

5) Repeat 10 times.

d) Quadriceps stretch

1) Using the opposite hand to your affected leg, hold the back of a chair or a table for support.

2) Stand a few centimeters away from this supporting chair/table.

3) Bend your affected leg at the knee and grab the foot with the free hand from behind.

4) Keep your back straight.

5) Pull on the foot from behind to stretch the quadriceps muscle.

6) Hold for 6 seconds.

7) Repeat 10 times.

Tip

Leaning your body forward slightly increases the tension on the quadriceps muscle.

13) Tibialis posterior exercises

a) Posterior tibialis tendon wall stretch

1) Place the affected foot on the wall, so that half of the foot is propped up against the wall, while the other half is on the ground.

2) With a straight knee lean forward, until a stretch is felt.

3) Hold for 15 seconds.

4) Release and repeat 10 times.

NB- This exercise can also be done with your knee bent.

b) Posterior tibialis tendon towel stretch

1) Sit on the ground, with both legs straight in front of you.

2) Grab a bathing towel at either end, with both hands.

3) Place the affected top half of the foot on the towel loop, maintaining the knee in a straight position.

4) Gently pull, until you feel a stretch.

5) Hold this position for 5 seconds

6) Release and repeat 10 times.

c) Toe off stretch

1) Sit in a chair, with both feet flat on the floor.

2) Raise the toes off the ground, keeping the heels on the ground.

3) Hold this stretch for 10 seconds.

4) Relax feet to the starting position.

5) Repeat this stretch 5 times, 3 times a day.

d) Posterior tibialis balancing stretch

1) Stand on the affected foot.

2) Balance with your eyes open for 2 minutes.

3) Then try balancing with your eyes closed.

4) Repeat 5 times.

e) Clapping feet stretch

1) Sit on a chair, with both of your legs hanging off the edge.

2) Place your feet close to each other, side by side.

3) While maintaining the side by side position of heels, actively bring the bottoms of your feet to face each other as if your feet are clapping.

4) Hold for 5 seconds.

5) Slowly return to the starting position and repeat 6-8 times.

14) Ankle tendonitis

a) Calf stretch (runner's stretch)

1) Stand with one foot in front of the other, both knees in a bent position.

2) Keep the back foot's heel on the ground, while you further bend the front knee forward, lifting its heel off the ground.

3) You will feel a stretch on the back leg.

4) Hold for 30 seconds and repeat with the other leg.

5) Make 5 switches.

b) Ankle roll

1) Sit on a chair, with the affected leg straight in front of you and above the ground.

2) Move the ankle in circles in a clockwise direction to make 10 revolutions.

3) Then repeat the process in a counterclockwise direction to make 10 revolutions.

4) Repeat 10-12 times.

c) Towel curls

1) Place a towel flat in front of a chair, on an uncarpeted surface.

2) Sit on the chair, and place your affected foot on top of the towel, with the heel touching the ground.

3) Pull the towel towards you by curling your toes over it to a grip, maintaining your heel position on the ground.

4) Repeat towel pulling 5 times.

Tip

Light weights can be placed on top of the towel to intensify the stretch.

d) Ankle inversion and eversion

1) Sit on a chair and cross your affected leg over the thigh of the normal leg to make a 4.

2) Grip the foot with the hand of the opposite side, placing your thumb below the foot and the other 4 fingers on top.

3) Gently move the foot counterclockwise on its side, as far as possible, holding the position for 10 seconds.

4) Switch the gripping on the foot, so that the thumb is on top of the foot, and the 4 fingers are below it. Curl the foot clockwise on its side as far as possible, and again, hold the position for 10 seconds.

5) Repeat 5 times.

15) Achilles physio exercises

a) Resistance band plantar flexion

1) While sitting on the ground, with the normal leg bent, stretch the affected leg straight in front of you.

2) Holding a resistance band on either end, with both hands, loop the band under the affected foot.

3) Pull the band with your hands to increase its resistance.

4) Point your foot away from you, slowly, over 4 seconds.

5) Repeat 10 times in 2 sets.

b) Eccentric heal drop

For the following exercise you require a step, like the ones used in aerobics.

1) Climb on top of the step.

2) Position your feet, so that half of the foot is over the edge of the step.

3) Slowly stand on tippy toes for 4 seconds.

4) Slowly lower your heels down, below the level of the step.

5) Do this 5-10 times.

Tip

This is a very hard exercise, ensure you are balanced well to avoid falling. Also, make sure your tendonitis healing stage allows this exercise to be done. Ask your physiotherapist.

c) Seated calf raise stretch

1) Sit on a chair, with your back against the back rest.

2) Raise your heels up, so that you are standing on tippy toes.

3) Hold the position for 10 seconds, then release your heels down.

4) Repeat 10 times in 2 sets.

d) Modified knee squat

1) Stand 2-3 inches away from the wall.

2) Bend your knees, until the kneecap touches the wall.

3) If you are very close to bend, step back a little and try again.

4) Hold the squat for 4 seconds.

5) Repeat 5 times.

e) Rocking stretch

1) Stand on both of your feet, applying more weight on the affected side.

2) Bend your knees to a walking or a running like position.

3) Lift the normal leg, with its knee still in a bent position.

4) Rock your body back and forth, while maintaining your back in a straight position.

5) Support yourself with the wall or chair, if required.

6) Rock for 30 seconds and rest.

7) Repeat 5 times.

f) Walking calf raise

This exercise can be done anywhere, as long as you are walking.

1) While you are walking, lift your heels off the ground.

2) Walk on tippy toes for 2 minutes, and switch to walk normally for 2 minutes.

3) Repeat this exercise over 12 minutes, so that you repeat tippy toeing for 2 minutes, 3 times.

16) Foot tendonitis stretches

a) Frozen can ball

1) Place the affected foot over a bottle of frozen water and/or a can of frozen beer or soda.

2) Roll the cold can back and forth, under your foot, for 2 minutes.

3) Rest for 2 minutes and repeat process 4 times.

NB- This exercise is better when done in the morning.

b) Alphabet stretch

1) Sit on a chair, with your affected leg hanging free.

2) With your ankle, write the letters of the alphabet in the air.

3) Imitate this writing with your foot pointed, to stretch the ankle, writing letters A to Z.

Tip

This stretch is good as a warm up before other exercises, as it involves the use of all muscles of the ankle and the foot.

c) Foot heel walking

1) Use your heels to walk for 30 seconds.

2) Stop and rest for 5 seconds.

3) Repeat heel walking for 30 more seconds.

NB- This exercise stretches your posterior leg muscles, ankle and foot.

d) Deep squats

1) Stand in a straight position, with your feet close together.

2) Bend down to a squatting position, lifting your heel off the ground as you do so.

3) Hold the position for 6 seconds.

4) Stand up and repeat 10 times.

e) Thera band inverter stretch

1) Place an elastic Thera band (found on Amazon.com) over your affected foot, holding each end of the band with your hands.

2) Step over the band, close to the affected ankle, with the normal foot, to increase tension on the elastic band.

3) Move your affected foot side to side, stretching as far as possible, repeat 10 times.

Index

Index

Dupuytren's contracture, 68

E

Elastin, 14
Elbow extensor muscle, 53
Endotenon, 16
Epicondyles, 55
Epitenon, 16
Erythrocyte sedimentation rate, 24
Extension, *39*
Extensor mechanism, 22
External rotation, 39
Extracellular matrix, 14

F

Faber's test, 75
Fasciae, 13
Fascicles., 16
Femur, 72
Fibroblasts, 29
Finkelstein test, 69
Flexion, 39
Full blood picture, 24

G

Glenoid fossa, 40
Glucosamine, *36*
Glycoproteins, 14
Golfer's elbow, 55
Golgi tendon organs, 18
Greater trochanter, 73
Groin, 72
Groin tendonitis, 75

H

Hamstring muscle, 73
Heart attack, 62

O

P

Q

R

S

Index

V

Vincula, 18

W

Watershed zone, 17

www.ingramcontent.com/pod-product-compliance
Lightning Source LLC
Chambersburg PA
CBHW060047210326
41520CB00009B/1299